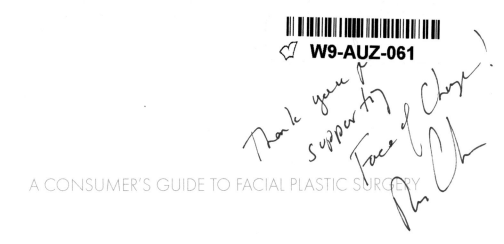

A CONSUMER'S GUIDE TO FACIAL PLASTIC SURGERY

YOUR
PLASTIC SURGERY
COMPANION

by:
Ross A. Clevens, M.D., FACS

with
David J. Mumford, Ed.D.

"Your facial plastic surgery experience
should be a journey, not merely a destination.
Make the most of your journey and enjoy your destination."

DEDICATION

In memory of my father, who remains with me every day.

To my mother, who told me I could do anything.

To my sons, a continuous fountain of amusement and reaffirmation that our future will always be greater than our past.

To my wife, the source of my strength, who has given me the most spectacular gift of my life … her unconditional love and her friendship.

Thank You,

Ross Clevens

ROSS A. CLEVENS, M.D., FACS

CREDENTIALS

EDUCATION

Yale University: B.S., summa cum laude, Phi Beta Kappa, Top five percent of class
Harvard Medical School: M.D., magna cum laude, Top three percent of class
Harvard University: M.P.H. in Health Policy and Management
Intern, Department of General Surgery, Beth Israel Hospital, Harvard Medical School
Resident, Department of Head and Neck Surgery, University of Michigan
Chief Resident, Department of Head and Neck Surgery, University of Michigan
Fellow, Facial Plastic and Reconstructive Surgery, University of Michigan

BOARD CERTIFICATIONS

American Board of Medical Examiners
American Board of Facial Plastic and Reconstructive Surgery
American Board of Otolaryngology-Head and Neck Surgery

HONORS AND AWARDS

Prize for Investigative Work, Columbia University College of Physicians and Surgeons
Leon Reznick Memorial Prize for Excellence in Research, Harvard Medical School

PROFESSIONAL AFFILIATIONS

Past President, Florida Society of Facial Plastic Surgeons
Fellow, American Academy of Facial Plastic and Reconstructive Surgery
Fellow, American Academy of Cosmetic Surgery
Fellow, American Society for Laser Medicine & Surgery
Fellow, American College of Surgeons
Diplomat, American Board of Facial Plastic and Reconstructive Surgery
Past President-Elect, Treasurer and Governor, Brevard County Medical Society

CHARITABLE INTERESTS

Founder, Face of Change,
A 501c(3) charitable entity responsible for providing medical care in the developing world,
and packaging nearly one million meals to feed local needy and hungry school children

TABLE OF **CONTENTS**

TABLE OF **CONTENTS**

CREDITS

Edited by:
Dr. Ross A. Clevens, M.D., FACS
Bernard Clevens
www.drclevens.com

Designed by:
Extremedia Group, Inc.
Some images used under license, provided by:
Shutterstock, iStock, Dreamstime

Published by:
Telemachus Press
www.telemachuspress.com

ISBN: 978-1-939337-07-8 (eBook)
ISBN: 978-1-939337-08-5 (Paperback)
ISBN: 978-1-939337-15-3 (Hardback)

2016.05.04

INTRODUCTION

When I first saw facial plastic surgery performed, it was love at first sight. Plastic surgery has an aura of excitement and creativity. It is surgery that adheres to the basic principles of anatomy and physiology but is deeply overlaid with psychosocial and personal concerns. This book has been many years in the making. It has taken twenty years to get to this point where I am able to share the knowledge and experience I have accumulated through the practice of the art and craft of facial plastic surgery. Like many authors, it has taken me years of thinking before daring to put pen to paper. From my point of view, this constitutes good writing: thinking first and writing second. Any other manner would be like putting the cart before the horse. All the thinking, the studying, the work and the experience finally rise to the surface here in this book, *"A Consumer's Guide to Facial Plastic Surgery: Your Plastic Surgery Companion"* Enjoy the journey!

Throughout the writing of this book, as in every day of the past twenty years of my surgical practice, I have kept my patient's well-being my primary concern. Patients entrust me as a facial plastic surgeon not only with their surgical care, but also with their most intimate fears and feelings. Patients discuss inadequacies, issues of body image and their deepest concerns with me. In facial plastic surgery, we try to restore each patient to the closest sense of normality as possible and to make each person look as good as possible. Our interactions with patients are typically brief but intense. With these thoughts in mind, my first and most important reason for writing this book is simply to inform. I want to share my knowledge with people, to help others discover the wonders of facial surgery and to aid them in navigating the confusing world of cosmetic surgery. This information is intended for general education purposes only and should not be relied upon as a substitute for professional and/or medical advice.

I want to give back to my patients and to my physician colleagues. I have been truly fortunate in my life to study in the world's finest academic institutions – Yale University, Harvard Medical School and The University of Michigan. Throughout my career I have also had the opportunity to work with some of the most competent and gifted talents in the field of facial plastic surgery as well as other areas of medicine. Now I want to do my part in sharing my knowledge with my past, present and future patients, my colleagues and the public general population as to what I believe is a very important, beneficial art for my fellow human beings – and that is not only to shape and reshape what is on the outside but also to enhance what is on the inside. I truly believe that just how a person perceives oneself starts from the outside but then most assuredly transcends into an inner discovery of self worth and beauty.

I have worked with literally thousands of patients throughout the course of my career, and every one of these patients has a unique story to tell. You can be assured that all patients have shared similar experiences throughout the process. Familiar patterns begin to develop: from the beginning of the process, which is an actual personal discovery of unique concern, transitioning into the next phase, which is a basic human need to know. Yes, curiosity sparks the desire to find out how to address our innermost concerns about our appearance.

In our experience at Clevens Face and Body Specialists, patients are most satisfied with their facial plastic surgery experience if they consider the following key question throughout their voyage:

"When we meet one year after your procedure has been performed, what has to have happened during that year for you to be happy with both the process and your result?"

At first glance, the 'answer' to this question appears self-evident. But as you ponder this question, give it some serious consideration before responding. Take a moment to re-read the question and think about what has to happen for you to be pleased with your outcome. It is a probing question that digs deep into your desired outcomes and motivations, as well as what you are hoping to accomplish during your facial surgery journey. Based upon our research into patient satisfaction with cosmetic surgery, we have developed a seven step unique process that guides our patients to success through the facial plastic surgery odyssey:

Step One – The Knowledge Builder™
Step Two – The Specialist Advantage™
Step Three – The Preparation and Reassurance Program™
Step Four – The Tailor Made Surgical Experience™
Step Five – The Nurturing Process™
Step Six – The Image Maximizer™
Step Seven – The Image Expander™

This book focuses upon this unique seven step process and elaborates upon the key elements within each step of the system.

Those first cautious steps into a cosmetic surgery center can be a very daunting experience. However, just like a baby, everyone has to take those first steps. As knowledge is built and confidence gained, momentum accelerates to a point where your preparation and reassurance encourages you. The tailor-made surgical experience is no longer faced with anxiety but with an educated firmness of conviction, courage and determination.

The nurturing process that follows is unique to everyone that undergoes facial plastic surgery. The commonality, however, is that everyone must sojourn through this phase. Your time for healing is also a time for learning. It is a time to recover from the physical aspects of the surgery as well as the psychosocial and emotional facets. Rest assured that all of our patients pass through this period of individual care,personal growth and adjustment.

But you will learn that the process does not stop after the surgery. In these pages of *"A Consumer's Guide to Facial Plastic Surgery: Your Plastic Surgery Companion"*, you will discover just how gratifying it is to take care of yourself and maximize the effects of your new image so you can enjoy the benefits of your facial plastic surgery experience. Proper diet and exercise are so important as you travel through this stage. A positive mindset emerges, as you are grateful for your renewed image. Surgery is not a destination, instead it is a journey to a new you – one with which you are more at ease and more pleased.

The Image Maximizer details surgical and non-surgical treatments that help to enhance your appearance and extend the results of your investment at your own pace. This information will help you to apply the knowledge you have built during your facial plastic surgery experience in the companionship of your friends, family and cosmetic surgery caregivers. You will learn about popular products and procedures that are producing remarkable results. The latest techniques and treatments are highlighted such as minimally invasive trends and the new laser technologies that are developing at lightning-fast speed. You will learn of various aesthetician services that are offered to enhance and, at times, even replace the need for surgery.

And remember, first and foremost, this book is about people. As unique as you are, you are not alone. Literally thousands of patients have walked through my doors and embarked on their own facial plastic surgery adventure. Each narrative is a secret treasure chest of human experience. Through this process, many patients have discovered something new about themselves that quite often became life changing.

So now, dear readers, I present to you, *"A Consumer's Guide to Facial Plastic Surgery: Your Plastic Surgery Companion"*, to Ensure Your Successful Facial Plastic Surgery Experience.

CHAPTER ONE
STEP ONE
THE KNOWLEDGE BUILDER

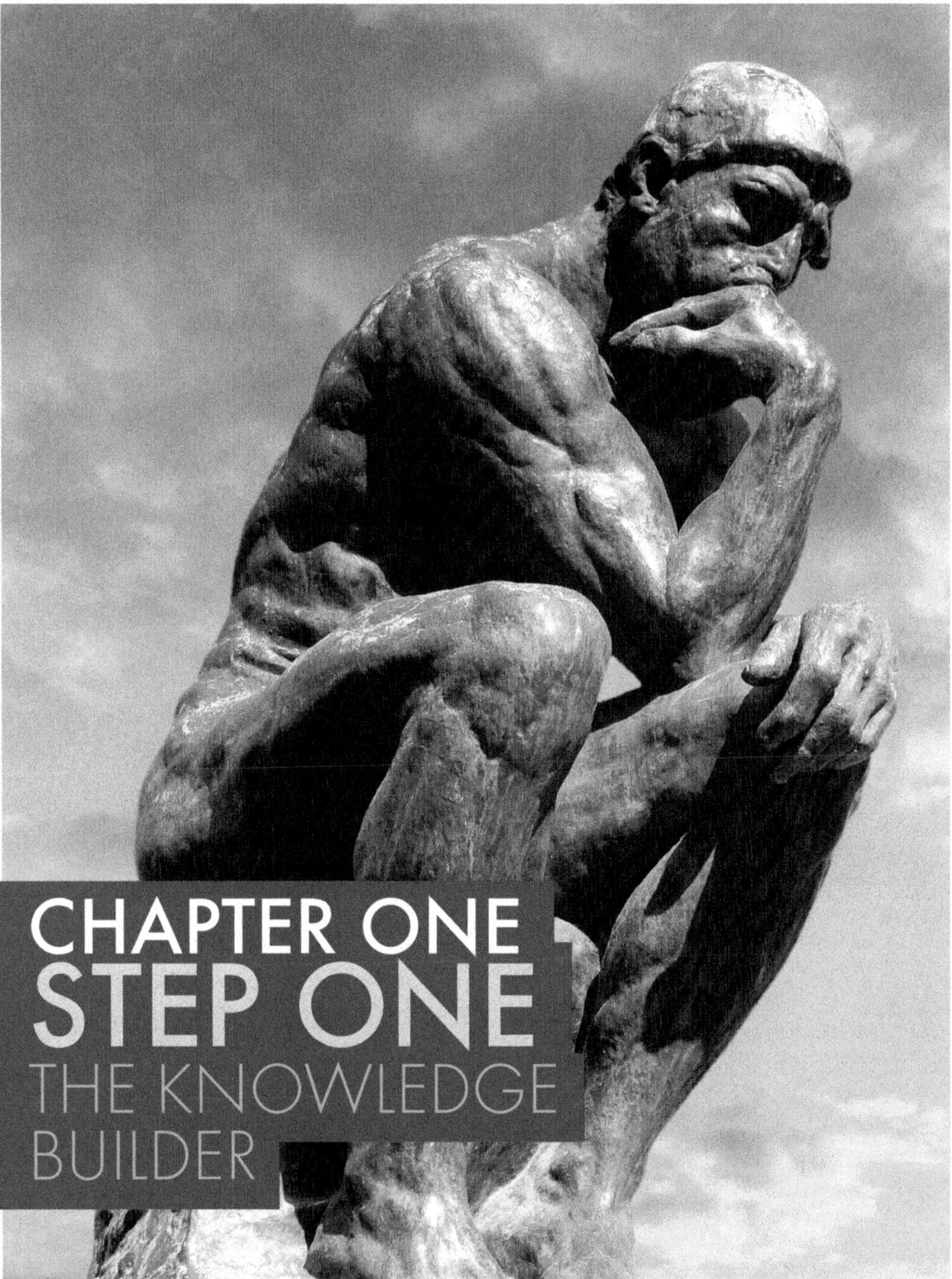

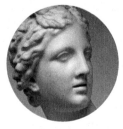

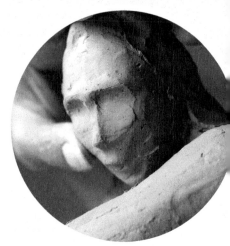

KNOWLEDGE IS POWER

id you know the term 'plastic surgery' comes from the ancient Greeks and refers to 'the art of modeling.' The artificial material that we know today as 'plastic' is not used in plastic surgery. Instead, the 'plastic' we refer to in plastic surgery is derived from the Greek plastikos, which means that something is supple, changeable or moldable. While Cosmetic Surgery is a relatively new field, the art and science of plastic surgery is centuries old. Records show that the first plastic surgery was performed in India nearly 2,500 years ago and the ancient Romans regularly partook in rudimentary beautification procedures several hundred years later.

If you look at the ancient history of most any culture, you can find records of people altering their bodies to look more desirable for their time. The need to fit in and to strive for the 'ideal' is a marker of being human. It is no wonder the field of plastic surgery continues to grow, expand, and develop. The drive to look better through plastic surgery is reflected in the enthusiasm for health, nutrition, wellness and fitness. It is a natural human desire.

Learning about the ancient societies can be insightful and interesting, but this process isn't about the Greeks or Egyptians. This process is about you! It is about providing you all the information you need in order to make a wise and informed decision about what you want to achieve with your own appearance.

When you embark on major life changes, it is important to get as much information as you can. This is especially true when you are looking to enhance your facial appearance. The first stage of this adventure consists of seeking factual information in order to learn everything that you can. This is really the most important part of the process towards cosmetic surgery. At our Center of Excellence, known as Clevens Face and Body Specialists, this stage is known as "The Knowledge Builder."

THE KNOWLEDGE BUILDER

b efore you even walk through the doors of a cosmetic surgery center, you have likely spent time researching procedures, looking at prospective surgeons and considering the world of possibilities.

Since you scheduled a consultation with the surgeon of your choosing means that you have sorted through all of the potential medical teams out there and decided that working with a facial plastic surgery specialist best fits your needs. Professional medical personnel understand how important this decision is to you, and you can be certain, the goal of your surgeon is to ensure that this decision becomes the best decision that you have ever made.

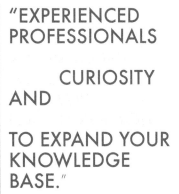

"EXPERIENCED PROFESSIONALS CURIOSITY AND TO EXPAND YOUR KNOWLEDGE BASE."

The Knowledge Builder process starts long before you ever schedule a consultation with a plastic surgeon, but it doesn't end with your consultation appointment either. You are encouraged to learn everything that you can about your potential procedure; as The Knowledge Builder is more than learning about the surgical process.

The Knowledge Builder also involves getting to know your surgical team and starting the process of developing key relationships. You will get to know the professionals that will attend you, and they will get to know you as well. The best patient is the most knowledgeable patient. Experienced professionals will welcome your curiosity and will encourage you to expand your knowledge base. This is a crucial part of your overall experience.

As a result, you can feel certain that from the moment you first step into a plastic surgery clinic for the first time, you have entered a center of excellence with the most highly competent and experienced medical staff. Fully qualified and caring staff members are prepared to receive you. They are there to help you with your unique and individual concerns.

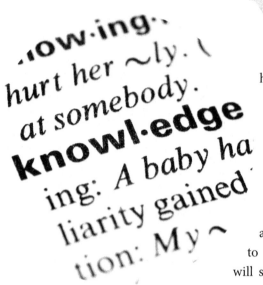

You have genuine concerns about the way you look, and these concerns affect how you feel about yourself. Since you have already done the research and have put a lot of thought into your situation, sharing this information with the right people is critical to your success.

Only by understanding what you want and need can the professionals start to build a level of communication that will serve you throughout the rest of your process.

And perhaps most importantly, good staff members understand that you need to develop a sense of trust before you are comfortable talking about your worries and fears.

During this part of the process, experts work hard to develop a connection with you and to create a strong relationship so they may gain the privilege of your trust. These experts who range from consultants to surgeons want you to feel comfortable and as relaxed as possible. Your honesty and openness is important to help us get the results you desire.

> PEOPLE WHO
> HAVE SOMETHING TO SAY AND CAN'T
> HAVE NOTHING TO SAY
> AND KEEP ON SAYING IT."
>
> *– Robert Frost*

Your key to gaining knowledge from your surgeon and his staff emerges from your candid communication with your team. It is important that you relate just how you feel about your present image. You need to be comfortable in sharing what is on your mind because this is how your team ensures your needs are met and your expectations are exceeded. Try asking yourself an important question. If you and your medical team were sitting down one year from today, what would you have hoped to accomplish together in order for you to be absolutely thrilled with your results?

Robert Frost, one of America's most revered poet laureates, once said, *"Half the world is composed of people who have something to say and can't and the other half who have nothing to say and keep on saying it."* It is our most sincere hope that you have a lot to say, and that you can and will say it. You deserve to be heard and a promise to listen should form the foundation of the patient-doctor relationship.

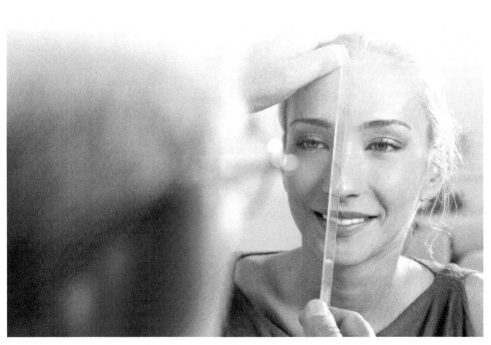

THE **AGING PROCESS**

YOUR FACE IS AN AMAZING CREATION.

IT IS COMPRISED OF AN INCREDIBLE PAIRED SET OF 44 PRECISE MUSCLES.

*t*he reality is that we are all going to age, and no matter how great our genes, eventually the signs of the unavoidable aging process are going to show on our bodies. The face is the first area that people look at when they see you. Aging in the face is going to say a lot more about your life than you might realize.

Whether we like it or not, people make assumptions, first impressions, and snap judgments about who you are and what we believe based on how you look. Research has shown that youthful, good-looking people are treated better, earn higher salaries and enjoy life more completely. Attractive people earn over $140,000 more than their 'average' looking peers over the course of a lifetime and at least 3-4% more annually. Attractive people are considered more influential and find more occupations available to them. This may seem unfair or superficial, but the unfortunate fact is that this is indeed true. It is important that your appearance truly matches how you feel and conveys the message that you want to send to the world. Looking and feeling better translates into greater personal and financial success.

Your face is an amazing creation. It is comprised of an incredible paired set of 44 precise muscles. These muscles are unlike any other muscles in the body. Whereas other muscles connect from bone to bone to move joints and limbs, facial muscles are unattached to bone and insert into the overlying skin. Their sole function is to create facial expressions that convey to your fellow man how you are feeling. Facial expression is a uniquely human characteristic that has evolved to allow nonverbal communication of emotion and intimacy.

It is remarkable that the human face can make over 7,000 different facial expressions. Imagine the complexity of emotion and feeling conveyed by this amazing anatomical array. And each face is completely unique. Look around you ... no two faces are alike! You should honor your face and recognize what a masterpiece it really is.

No matter how much you love the way you look, the aging process is inevitable for each and every one of us. As each decade passes, there will be certain changes that affect your face, neck, and skin. What basic changes should you expect to see as you age and what cosmetic procedures might be able to help you curb the signs of aging? Let's explore your options in the following paragraphs.

	ISSUE	SOLUTION
IN YOUR 20'S	Sun Damage	Sunblock with SPF Greater than 30
	Fine Wrinkles	Begin Doctor Supervised Skin Care Regimen for Life
	Early Changes in Brow, Crow's Feet and Lips	Injectable Fillers and Relaxers
	Concerns with Nasal Profile	Rhinoplasty or Nose Job
	Protruding Ears	Otoplasty or Ear Pinning
	Weak Chin or Cheeks	Chin or Cheek Implants
IN YOUR 30'S	Drooping Eyelids	Eyelid Procedure
	Fine Lines	Skin Resurfacing
	Wrinkles around Mouth	Injectables
	Skin Laxity	Laser or RF Skin Tightening
	Sun Damaged Skin	Fractional Laser Skin Resurfacing
IN YOUR 40'S	Frown Lines	Brow Lift
	Deepening of Wrinkles	Injectables
	Crow's Feet	Eyelid Procedure
IN YOUR 50'S	Pouches in Cheeks	Cheek Implants
	Double Chin	Facelift
	Jaw Line Sagging	Facelift
	Eyebrow Sagging	Eyelid Procedure
IN YOUR 60'S	Hooded Eyelids	Eyelid Procedure
	Loss of Elasticity	Facelift
	Forehead Lines	Brow Lift
	Deep Wrinkles	Injectables
	Neck Skin Sagging	Facelift

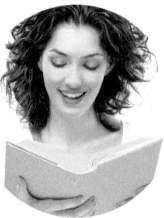

EXPLORATORY
QUESTIONS

oming in for your consultation involves learning more about your potential surgical procedure as well as begins the process of building rapport. Naturally, you will likely have plenty of questions about process, procedure, and the like, that we will discuss later. Before we explore these details, we want to talk about the specific reasons behind your plan for cosmetic surgery. Take a moment and consider the following questions:

> What is it that bothers you about your appearance?
>
> How is this concern affecting your life?
>
> How do you think surgery will address the problem?
>
> Will surgery change your feelings about yourself?
>
> How do you think your new image will make your life better?
>
> How long of a recovery time do you have available?
>
> Are you seeking a surgical or non-surgical solution?
>
> What is your budget?
>
> What anxieties or fears do you have?
>
> What needs to happen in order for you to be happy with your outcome and during your journey?

Questions like these are extremely important. Sharing your thoughts about these questions with your facial plastic surgeon will help your team better understand what you might be expecting surgery to do for you. The answers to these questions will also help to determine the best course of action. And, most importantly, the answers to these questions might just give you a better idea of what you really want.

At this point in your journey, we at Clevens Face and Body Specialists encourage our patients to start a journal. Consider this journal your official cosmetic procedure diary. It is the one place where you can keep track of your thoughts and feelings about your procedure as well as the process. By writing in a journal you can start to find clarity around your situation. It is a place where you can intimately express your issues, worries, fears, and excitement. This can help you confidentially express your questions and concerns to your surgeon and your team, and communicate exactly what you want and what you are feeling.

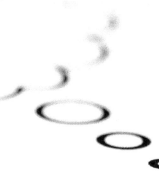

SURGICAL JOURNAL

CHECKLIST OF QUESTIONS ANSWERED

*i*f you read the above questions and don't yet have clear answers, or any answers at all, we encourage you to write these questions down in your surgical journal. In fact, even if you do have clear answers we recommend that you write these questions down and give some time and thought to the answers. Make this the first thing you do with your journal. Even if your answers seem obvious right now, write them out anyway. You might be surprised by what comes up.

You may also want to start a photographic journal that can also be used for pasting photos, images, and other items that relate to how you might want to change your appearance. This album might include photos of yourself, perhaps photos that expose what concerns you. Many patients find that collecting images from when they were younger helps them to collect and organize their thoughts about what they want to correct. Some patients will also clip pictures of celebrities and athletes who have characteristics that they are hoping to emulate. In considering rhinoplasty (nasal contouring surgery), as an example, it is very common for folks to cut out pictures of noses they like and do not like in order to communicate their wishes more clearly to their surgeon.

Like all diaries, your facial plastic surgery journal may be a private place where your thoughts, fears and desires can be stored. By keeping all of your information in one place you can more easily show us what you want and express how you are feeling.

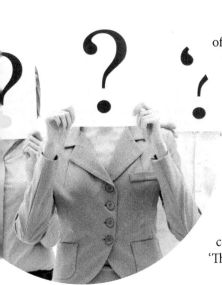

he next thing you should do in your journal is to create a list of questions for your surgeon and team to answer. We refer to this as a 'checklist of questions.' This will help you to remember all of the issues that you want to have addressed when we meet. By having everything in one place it will be easier for you to share what is important and to have all of your questions answered.

The goal of facial cosmetic surgery is to create a happy and satisfied patient at the end of the journey. The definition of satisfaction varies from one patient to the next and not all patients would answer a set of questions in the same way. This is the individuality of each person's unique set of concerns, which we try to uncover as part of the 'The Knowledge Builder' phase of your odyssey.

A CHECKLIST OF QUESTIONS

nytime you are getting a procedure done, seek a well trained and board certified surgeon in the proper area of expertise. Doctors certified by the American Board of Facial Plastic and Reconstructive Surgery (www.abfprs.org) have completed rigorous training lasting from five to seven years beyond college and medical school specializing in facial, head and neck surgery and have passed a comprehensive certifying exam. Such surgeons are uniquely qualified to perform facial cosmetic and reconstructive surgery.

Surgeons certified by the American Board of Plastic Surgery have also completed extensive training in plastic surgery. Plastic surgeons commonly focus on all aspects of plastic and reconstructive surgery, not only facial surgery but also surgery of the breast, body and extremities.

SEEK A WELL TRAINED.
AND BOARD CERTIFIED SURGEON
IN THE PROPER AREA OF EXPERTISE

You will likely have a set of your own questions that you will want answered, but here is a checklist that we recommend patients consider to ensure they have the answers before moving forward with any surgeon:

Is what you want exactly what you need?
Does my surgeon specialize in the sort of procedure I am considering?
How often does my surgeon perform the procedure that interests me?
Is surgery the answer or are there alternatives?
If surgery is the answer, then what will my image be afterwards?
Do you have that computer imaging technique that I've seen advertised so much in the newspaper and on television?

Also keep in mind the specific questions connected to the procedure, before, during, and after:

Where will the actual surgery take place: in a hospital, in the clinic?
What kind of preparation will I have to make at home and at work before the surgery?
How long will the surgery itself take?
Will I have to undergo anesthesia, and if so, what kind?
Will I be in pain?
What kinds of medication will I have to take before and after?
Will I have any side effects and what are the risks of complications?
Will I need some kind of at-home care?
When will I be able to go back to my normal activities?
When can I go back to work?

The next questions to consider are related to money and payment:

If surgery is the answer, then how much will it cost?
Will I have to pay for this in one lump sum or can I pay over a period of time?
Will my insurance cover this? How can I find out?
What is included in the fee and what is not included?
Are anesthesia and facility fees included or extra?
Will I need a nurse after surgery to help take care of me and how much does this cost?

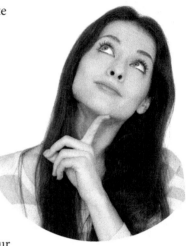

ll of these are serious and legitimate questions that rightfully concern every patient. Because insurance does not include most facial cosmetic surgery procedures, you will need to pay out of pocket in all likelihood. Do not be bashful about asking questions related to cost and what is and is not included in your cost estimate. You deserve clarity up front as to your financial investment. Listed above are some of the more common questions that your surgeon and his staff should address during your consultation. But there will be many more. Just remember to write all of your questions down in your journal and bring them up during your consultations.

You need to be informed and educated throughout your process. Our philosophy at Clevens Face and Body Specialists is that the best patient is the well-educated patient. We truly believe that the more prepared you are for your first meeting with our team of professionals, the less anxiety you will have as you start to move forward towards your procedure. This philosophy is what The Knowledge Builder is all about. You need to feel comfortable and at ease with the surgeon and his attending staff. When you have comfort and ease, you will feel more self-assured and confident that what you are doing is the absolute right thing to do. Knowledge is power.

"DO NOT BE ASKING QUESTIONS

As we move forward in this chapter you will see questions in bold. These are questions that you should answer before your consultation appointment. This is another place where you should write these questions down and take your time in answering them. Bring your answers with you to your consultation. This will help the process go smoother and ensure that you have given your undivided attention to the questions. Many patients feel that their concerns are not fully addressed in a single visit to the doctor. Questions arise after their visit. We have found that many patients return in person for a second consultation to clarify their concerns. Other patients email or call to be certain that all of their questions are answered.

As part of the Knowledge Builder process, patients are encouraged to return to make certain that their questions are fully addressed to their complete satisfaction before scheduling their procedure.

WHAT ARE
YOUR EXPECTATIONS?

Coming into your consultation with your journal is a great first step. This will help you to have all of your thoughts and ideas in one place. This is very important because one of the first things the staff will want to know is what your expectations are for your facial surgery.

Unfortunately, there is a lot of false and unrealistic information about plastic surgery. Inconsistent information can be found on the internet, in different forms of media and even in some printed literature. For the first time, prospective facial plastic surgery patients are facing a barrage of infomercials from national plastic surgery chains that have unfortunately brought fast food quality to the art of plastic surgery. Too often patients come to their consultations with a fantasy of what their lives will be like after their procedure is completed. These fantasies have been influenced by unreliable, and often wrong, information. If it sounds too good to be true, then it probably is.

Too often, people believe that cosmetic surgery will cure their depression, help them find true love, make them famous, or make them rich. The reality is that none of these things is true. And if any of these claims are part of your expectations, then you are seeking plastic surgery for the wrong reasons. You should consider facial plastic surgery for yourself -- to help you feel better about yourself and to make you look as good as you feel. Facial plastic surgery should be for you, so you feel better about yourself and for no one else. Because there is so much incorrect information available, we believe it is important to create a realistic picture of what you can expect from your procedure. The best way to avoid disappointment in your surgical outcome is to have a clear and realistic idea of what plastic surgery can do for you. Again, knowledge is power. When you share what you want, experienced professionals are able to give you a clear picture of what is possible and what they can do to help you get there. If you do discover some misconceptions during the consultation, the goal of the medical team should be to educate you on what can be expected from your surgical procedure and give you a more accurate vision of reality.

Your facial plastic surgeon and his staff should be straightforward in informing you, both in conversation and in written form, precisely what plastic surgery can and cannot do. Knowledge is power and with a little help you will grow confident in making an educated decision on what is best for your future.

The American Academy of Facial Plastic and Reconstructive Surgery (www.aafprs.org) has a very reliable and accurate website. This site also features brief descriptions and videos of the main procedures in facial plastic surgery (www.aafprs.org/patient/pro-cedures/proctypes.html). The Clevens Face and Body Specialists site (www.drclevens.com) is another reliable source of information for prospective patients.

WHY ARE **YOU** DOING IT?

hy do you want plastic surgery? This might seem like a silly question, of course, because you simply want to change your look. But this is actually one of the most important questions that is asked during your consultation. It is important to assess your intention behind seeking plastic surgery. I often ask my patients, "Why now?"

It is imperative that you are seeking surgery solely for your own reasons and not for someone else's or with a different ulterior motive. If you are looking to get plastic surgery because someone else in your life wants you to do it, then it is likely that there are underlying problems that the surgery will not be able to solve.

Getting surgery for someone else is never the right answer. If you are seeking a cosmetic procedure to satisfy someone other than yourself, then disappointment is likely and we will encourage you to look at other options rather than a cosmetic procedure.

Plastic surgery is a gift to yourself because you have earned the privilege and because you deserve it.

PLASTIC SURGERY IS A GIFT TO YOURSELF BECAUSE YOU DESERVE IT.

WHAT ARE YOUR
POSSIBLE OPTIONS?

fter discussing your reasons and hopes for your cosmetic procedure, we will then review the possible outcomes and the options that are available to you. When you have a clear picture of what the end results might be, you will have a better idea as to whether plastic surgery is truly what you want at this time.

As briefly discussed before, there are many misconceptions as to what plastic surgery can do. It is important that you understand that you will not just wake up after surgery, look in the mirror, and instantaneously see your face magically transformed. There is a period of healing and recovery before your final outcome will be seen and 'the new you' is apparent. This aspect of facial plastic surgery is discussed in greater detail later in the book and in your personal consultation.

It is also important that you are psychologically prepared for the results of your procedure. Counting on the successful outcome of your facial surgery, you will want to give some thought as to how you will respond to yourself, your friends, and your family. Looking into the mirror and seeing a different reflection looking back at you can be a challenging experience. This is often a reflection of a younger looking you ... perhaps as you looked 10-15 years ago. Or, it might be a version of you without some troubling attribute such as a crooked nose, a hump on your nose or protruding ears. Regardless of your concerns, there will be a new you in the mirror.

You might think that seeing an improved version of your face won't be a big deal, but many people take a while to grow accustomed to their new appearance. Even when subtle changes are made they may seem like major changes to you. No one knows your face like you do, and even the tiniest adjustment can appear totally transformative when you look in the mirror. Your new reflection may not appear exactly as you anticipated, but it should be a refreshing improvement that may take some time to get used to. Rest assured though, you will look better, not different.

*f*amily members might not be as supportive to the process as you would like them to be. Often patients try and hide their procedure from their spouse, but we strongly encourage involving your family in this important decision. Having support from your loved ones is critical. Being honest with them is going to help you feel more secure and at peace with your decision. Hopefully, you have shared your motivation with your family members and they value your decision. This openness and understanding calms the waters for smooth sailing.

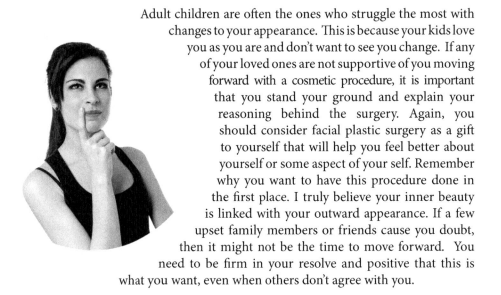

Adult children are often the ones who struggle the most with changes to your appearance. This is because your kids love you as you are and don't want to see you change. If any of your loved ones are not supportive of you moving forward with a cosmetic procedure, it is important that you stand your ground and explain your reasoning behind the surgery. Again, you should consider facial plastic surgery as a gift to yourself that will help you feel better about yourself or some aspect of your self. Remember why you want to have this procedure done in the first place. I truly believe your inner beauty is linked with your outward appearance. If a few upset family members or friends cause you doubt, then it might not be the time to move forward. You need to be firm in your resolve and positive that this is what you want, even when others don't agree with you.

Overall you must want to have the surgery because of you and you alone. What others think shouldn't really matter, but you will still need to deal with the reactions and opinions of the people in your life. Being prepared for these reactions is going to be important to making the final decision about whether or not moving forward with your surgery is right for you.

When thinking about your physical changes after the cosmetic procedure, here are some important questions to ask yourself:

> How will you plan on assimilating back into your circle of friends with your new look?
>
> Will they like the results, will they not, will they be indifferent?
>
> Will you be prepared to handle the responses, come what may?
>
> What if your friends are not supportive of the new you?
>
> Do you have the confidence to appreciate the change?
>
> What if your reflection is improved, but its not quite exactly what you had hoped for?

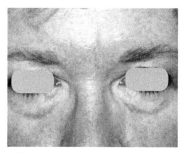 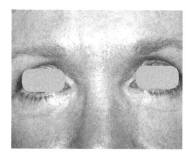

Actual Patient;
Eyebrow Lift

Before

After

After seeing some images of possible outcomes from your cosmetic procedure, it is important to ask yourself these two questions:

Are the end results that we discuss what you really want?
Are the end results what you really expect or do you have further doubts?

If you have doubts, or if the outcome isn't what you expected, this is important information for you and for your surgeon and his team to know. You can discuss other alternatives to surgery that might be more conducive to achieving your desired result. There are other ways to solve certain facial aesthetic concerns. If you are apprehensive about whether or not you are ready for a surgical procedure, you can look at some of the non-surgical solutions with your surgical team. The bottom line is if you are not totally ready and 100 percent sure, then the surgery should not happen.

Minimal or non-invasive procedures are becoming more common. Certain creams and sunblocks, moisturizers, lasers, Botox and other injectables are among the less invasive options that might be a better fit for you. If you still want to make changes to your appearance but have doubts about the surgical process, we will happily explore these other options with you. At the current pace of innovation, these alternative options increase in number practically every day.

THE BOTTOM LINE IS IF YOU ARE NOT TOTALLY READY AND 100 PERCENT SURE, THEN THE SURGERY SHOULD NOT HAPPEN.

LET'S GO TO THE
COMPUTER

odern technology has given us the ability, through computer programs, to create an image of what you might look like after your cosmetic procedure. The results we are able to get from these computer programs are remarkably accurate. Facial Cosmetic Surgery Imaging is truly a modern miracle. The technology allows you to view yourself before and after the cosmetic surgery is completed.

Let's say, for example, that you are considering having your eyes done. The images on the computer screen can show you just what you will look like after surgery addresses your dark circles, excess skin, or the bags underneath your eyes. With a few simple clicks of the computer program, the imagery will immediately display what the art of plastic surgery can do to sculpt younger looking eyes. The same process can be applied to all other aspects of the face: for example, shape a new nose, contour the chin, rejuvenate the neck, or even erase unsightly wrinkles caused by the passage of time, smoking or excess sun exposure.

Facial Cosmetic Surgery Imaging can educate you on what will be done and exactly how the surgery will be performed to create the best desired results for your unique image. This program can give you a visualization of your predicted results. Armed with this visual depiction of your results, you will have details of the best path towards obtaining the results that you want.

Facial Cosmetic Surgery Imaging is an important educational tool. Although actual results may vary owing to the complexity and uniqueness of the human body, imaging creates a forum where the surgeon can interact with you and discuss the possible variations of the results. For example, the surgeon may image a patient seeking rhinoplasty (nasal contouring) who is also wondering whether or not to consider a chin implant. The surgeon can create two 'after' images, one with rhinoplasty and chin implant and one with rhinoplasty alone. This enables the patient to visualize the results of both versions. As we've remarked already in this book, the goal of cosmetic surgery is to create a happy patient -- one who is pleased with his or her surgical outcome. Facial Cosmetic Surgery Imaging enhances patient satisfaction because it helps your outcome on the computer match the vision that you have in your mind's eye.

VISIA DIGITAL SKIN CARE ANALYSIS

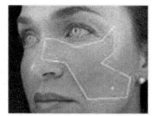

Spots (85%)

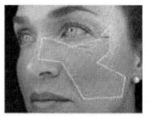

Pores (98%)

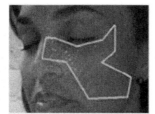

Porphyrins (29)

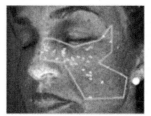

Wrinkles (75%)

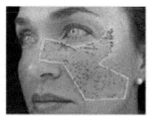

Evenness (89%)

UV Spots (32)

long with the Facial Cosmetic Surgery Imaging program your professional team can also use the VISIA Digital Skin Care Analysis. This program is cutting edge and uses video imaging that will show you the specifics of skin damage, both on the surface and deep beneath the skin. This unique look below the skin's surface can determine to what degree the skin has been damaged, thereby allowing your skin caregiver to ascertain with great accuracy the proper treatment for any particular skin disorder you might be dealing with.

VISIA analysis uses unique digital imaging techniques that unveil the underlying condition of your skin. VISIA reveals the degree of sun damage, pigment changes, spider vein formation and skin texture and quality. Many cosmetic facial surgery centers use VISIA technology to help select the methods of skin care, non-surgical solutions, and surgical procedures that are best suited to the needs of your skin. Imperfections of the skin such as lines, brown spots and sun damage occur at different levels of the skin. Some changes occur deeper in the skin at the level of the dermis, while others affect only the surface of the skin or the epidermis.

Technologies such as VISIA analysis help to determine at which level within the skin the changes have occurred. With the knowledge gained from VISIA imaging, the appropriate treatment method can be fine tuned to target the site of damage.

THE SCIENCE
OF BEAUTY

did you know there is a scientific equation that reveals what people consider beautiful? It has been proven that an even and symmetrical face is considered to be more beautiful. The more symmetrical a person's face, the more appealing that person is to the opposite sex. Recalling notions put forth by the ancient Greeks, research confirms that balanced facial features are considered more beautiful by observers. Symmetry is perhaps the most important ingredient in human impression of beauty. The good news is that symmetry can often be created with surgical means.

There is a certain amount of physical beauty that can be measured. There is a mathematical equation that can be used to measure the symmetry and determine how attractive your face actually is. Using this system, if one or two things are adjusted in an unattractive face, it suddenly becomes attractive. Very little change is needed to totally transform how someone is viewed. These are subtle changes indeed.

It has been proven that the following features comprise an attractive female face:

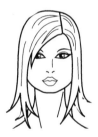

Short upper lip
High cheekbones
Small nose
Short distance between the chin and mouth
Large eyes, widely spaced apart
Fine jawline
Petite chin

A man's face on the other hand seems to be held to a different set of beauty standards. Here is a listing of what is considered attractive in a male face:

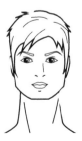

Heavy brows
Full head of hair
Prominent chin
Strong jawline
Rectangular face shape
Deep set eyes

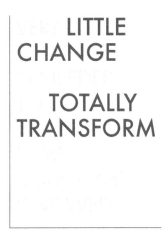

O f course, very few individuals on the planet have a perfectly symmetrical face … at least without some help. Naturally, there always will be some asymmetries between the left and right sides of our faces; this is what makes each of us appear unique as individuals. During your consultation, your facial plastic surgeon should examine the symmetry of your face and see what can be done to bring more evenness to your look.

It is believed that much of your psychological well-being is connected to your sense of self-esteem. The creator of modern plastic surgery, Jacques Joseph, said that self-esteem is enhanced when the facial features are in harmony. So much of beauty and attractiveness is based upon the balance and interplay of facial features. A weak chin or a high, sloping brow makes our nose look prominent. A down-turned corner of the mouth creates the impression of anger or bitterness. We look tired if our lids and brows are droopy. Society places such a large emphasis on the way we look. The way that we look sends messages to other people about who we are. The way we look gives people clues to how we feel and even what our aspirations are. In certain cases, plastic surgery helps our outside appearance mirror our inside feelings.

It used to be that only the wealthy, famous, and elite could get plastic surgery, but this is no longer the case. Advancements in the field and growing interest in cosmetic procedures have made it possible for people of any background to be able to get cosmetic procedures.

Whether we want to believe it or not, people who are considered attractive by these standards tend to have an easier way getting through the world. People are more likely to help out someone they consider beautiful rather than someone they consider plain. This has been proven in studies time and time again. Psychologists say that beautiful people get better jobs, earn more money, get better service, and even have better sex lives.

"Beautiful People" does not have to be a term that is referring to someone else. Anyone can be one of the "Beautiful People." All it takes is a little commitment from you to make the change.

LITTLE CHANGE

TOTALLY TRANSFORM

SKIN TYPE AND SURGERY

Your skin type, ethnicity, skin color, and the texture of your skin will all have a bearing on how you will age and the major issues that you might be facing as time goes on. Here is a basic breakdown of the different skin types, how they age, and their significance in cosmetic procedures. Of course, it is important to keep in mind that you are an individual and each person is going to be different. This is just a starting point.

ANGLO-SAXON { FAIR COMPLECTED WITH RED HAIR }

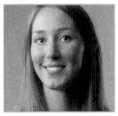

Individuals with this background tend to have red hair, blue or green eyes, freckled skin that is sensitive. With sun exposure, their skin burns and never tans. Skin cancer and sun damage are common with marked sun sensitivity. People who are fair-skinned have several benefits that will help them with cosmetic procedures. The skin drapes easily, which allows more precise changes to be made. Scars are usually small, heal easily, and are mostly unnoticeable. Swelling with this type of skin is minimal, but bruising may be more obvious. The challenges with this skin type are that the signs of aging will appear earlier than with any other skin type. They are more prone to sun damage. Fine wrinkles may be more difficult to remove and any irregularities in the face or on the skin are much more obvious against the fine white complexion.

NORTHERN EUROPEAN { FAIR COMPLECTED WITH BLONDE HAIR }

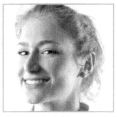

People who are fair-skinned with blond hair are very similar to the Anglo-Saxon type of skin. They tend to have blue or green eyes and sensitive skin that burns rather than tans with sun exposure. Skin cancer and sun damage are also common with marked sun sensitivity. The skin tends to be thin, which means that it is easy to manipulate. Incisions disappear easily and blend within the skin. Swelling with this type of skin is minimal, but bruising may occur. The signs of aging are going to be obvious early and deep wrinkles may form die to sun sensitivity.

AFRICAN { DARK COMPLECTED WITH DARK HAIR AND EYES }

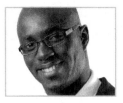

This skin type shows the signs of aging at the latest point. The skin is resistant to sun damage and skin cancer is rare. Fine wrinkles typically never form. Swelling from surgical procedures may last a while but bruising is less common. Scarring may become thickened with this type of dark complexion. Certain sites tend to form thickened scars, but again, facial incisions tend to heal much better than non-facial sites. There is also a greater risk of pigmentation issues and the cartilage isn't easily manipulated. Attentive care during and after surgery improves healing of the incisions.

CENTRAL EUROPEAN { OLIVE COMPLECTED WITH DARK HAIR }

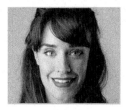

Individuals of this ethnogeographic background tend to have thicker and more oily skin. The skin is less sensitive to the sun. It tends to tan rather than burn. Hair and eyes are commonly dark. Sun damage and skin cancer is less common. This skin type is more protected from the sun and signs of aging appear a little bit later in life. Incisions are often thin and easy to hide. The structure of bones and cartilage is stronger and often easy to work with. People with this skin type often run into pigmentation. There can be unwanted blotchiness of the skin with areas of lightening and darkening. Pale incisions may be more obvious than with some of the lighter skin tones.

SOUTH EUROPEAN HISPANIC, ASIAN PACIFIC
{ ETHNOGEOGRAPHIC SKIN AND HAIR PIGMENTATION }

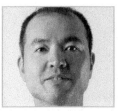

The signs of aging will appear much later with this skin type. Fine lines and wrinkling are less with this type of skin owing the protection from the sun gained by its pigmentation. On the other hand the skin tends to be thicker, which means that it is more resistant to lifting during surgical processes. Swelling tends to last longer with this skin type and scarring may be thicker, darker, and more obvious. There are certain precautions we must take at the time of surgery and in the after-care to ensure optimal healing. It is fortunate that facial incisions tend to heal much better than non-facial sites.

SOUTH ASIAN, INDIAN
{ DARK COMPLECTED WITH THICKER, MORE OILY SKIN }

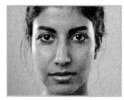

The signs of aging come on much later than with most of the other lighter skin types. Cancer of the skin is very rare with this skin type. The cartilage with this skin type is resistant to surgical manipulation and tends to droop with aging. Thickened scars may occur and swelling after surgical procedures can last longer than in fine skinned individuals. At the time of surgery we exercise great care in the placement and closure of incisions to improve the outcome. There are special care techniques after surgery that can improve healing. Again, it is fortunate that facial incisions tend to heal much better than non-facial sites and keloid scarring is rare on the face.

HOW WILL YOU PREPARE
FOR YOUR FIRST VISIT
WITH YOUR FACIAL PLASTIC SURGEON?

b y the time you schedule your individual consultation with your facial plastic surgeon, you will have already taken the very important first step towards your successful facial surgery - talking to the clinic staff.

Your next step will be to talk to the surgeon personally, allowing him or her to establish exactly what can be done for you and to clarify your vision of how you want to look. Tools such as your journal, computerized video imaging and VISIA imaging will help you get the most out of your consultation.

THE DECISION

PLASTIC SURGERY

WHAT IS BEST FOR YOU.

In order for your consultation to be successful there are some things that you need to do in preparation for your visit with the facial surgeon.

It takes a lot to walk in the front door of a facial plastic surgeon's office. The decision to seek facial plastic surgery is about having courage to stand up and do what is best for you. Getting surgery is a big step that will change your life. When you feel better about yourself you will start living a fuller life.

A staff member's desire is to make you feel as comfortable as possible, but your first meeting with a surgeon might make you nervous. The whole process can be quite stressful, confusing, and even frustrating.

Many patients get so nervous during their initial meeting that they forget everything they want to say and all the questions they want to ask. We have found among our patients that this is a remarkably common experience.

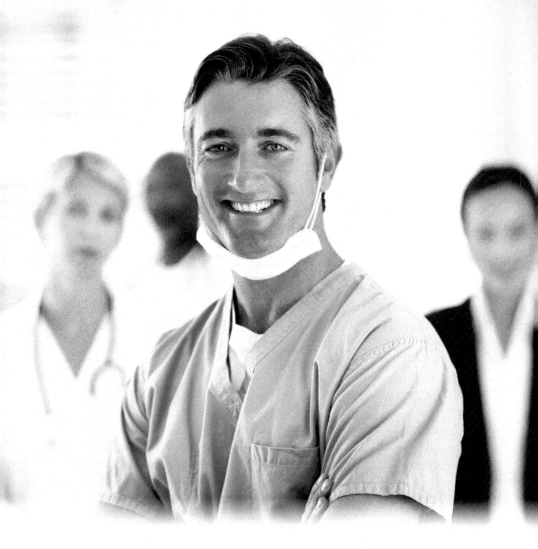

Having your surgical journal (or even this book, see the notes sections at the end of each chapter and on page 224) with you is the best way to prepare for this meeting. Answering all of the questions that we have already outlined and having these questions in your journal is important.

Having your checklist of the questions that you want to have answered is going to make your consultation smooth, easy, and productive.

And lastly, having a clear idea of what you want out of the cosmetic procedure will help you and your surgeon see where you are headed and determine how to get there.

Being prepared before you go for the consultation will help diminish any anxieties that you might be feeling because you will know that you are getting all of the information you need.

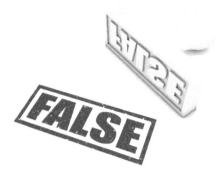

MYTHS AND LEGENDS
OF PLASTIC SURGERY

a s we have said before, there is a lot of false information available about plastic surgery: what it is, what it can do, and how it can change your appearance. Continuing with the idea that knowledge is power, here are some of the plastic surgery myths and the truth and the reality behind them.

MYTH: YOU CAN TELL WHEN SOMEONE HAS HAD "WORK DONE."

REALITY: No doubt you can flip through a magazine or watch a Hollywood event and try to guess who has had work done. We have even heard of people making a game out of it. The truth is that many more people have had cosmetic procedures than you can tell have had them. It is the 'bad' or 'overdone' plastic surgery that is obvious. Most people don't want to make it look obvious that they have had plastic surgery, which is our goal. We want to help you look better, not different. Modern and sophisticated plastic surgery looks quite natural, like turning back the hands of a clock with a magic wand.

MYTH: YOU CAN ONLY GET ONE PROCEDURE AT A TIME.

REALITY: Many patients undergo several treatments at the same time. This is not only easier for you as far as recovery time, but it is also less expensive. When you get a brow lift and an eyelid procedure at the same time you only have to cover the costs of the surgical room, anesthesiologist, and medications once. Plus, the recovery time for both of these surgeries is going to be shorter than if you did each of them as a separate procedure broken up over time. Performing complementary procedures at the same time is not only more efficient in terms of cost and time, but also creates more natural and pleasing results. It can look unnatural to rejuvenate one part of your face yet leave an adjacent region unimproved.

MYTH: PLASTIC SURGERY CAN CHANGE ANYTHING WITH YOUR FACE OR BODY THAT YOU DON'T LIKE.

REALITY: This is one of the harsher myths that prevail. Facial plastic surgeons can't totally transform your look. They still have to work with your underlying facial structure and that can't always be changed. If you have a specific look that you want to create, surgeons may or may not be able to do that. That is exactly why they go over the realities of cosmetic surgery during consultations. This is so you know what to expect and what is realistic. Previewing video imaging that digitally modifies your appearance to simulate the results of surgery can be helpful in establishing expectations.

MYTH: PLASTIC SURGERY ISN'T 'REAL' SURGERY.

REALITY: Plastic surgery is, in fact, real surgery and should not be undertaken lightly. Yes, there are many cosmetic benefits to the process, but there are also risks to having plastic surgery performed. It is important to take into consideration your overall health and well-being for surgery and your preparedness for your procedure. Anytime you are getting a procedure done, seek a well-trained and board certified surgeon in the proper area of expertise. Doctors certified by the American Board of Facial Plastic and Reconstructive surgery have completed rigorous training in facial, head and neck surgery and have passed a comprehensive certifying exam. Such surgeons are uniquely qualified to perform facial cosmetic surgery.

MYTH: PLASTIC SURGERY LEAVES NO SCARS.

REALITY: During a cosmetic surgery procedure, incisions are made. It is impossible to make incisions without some sort of scarring taking place. This is why facial plastic surgeons are required to go through so much training and schooling before they can perform these procedures. Yes, there will be scars, but most often they are hidden or placed where they are not noticeable. The face is blessed with a remarkable capacity for healing, more so than any other part of the body. Facial incisions generally heal very nicely and should not be obvious after your procedure.

MYTH: ONLY WOMEN GET PLASTIC SURGERY.

REALITY: Although the majority of plastic surgery recipients are women, men now seek appearance enhancement in much higher numbers than in the past. Research has shown that men desire aesthetic improvement as much as women do and that cosmetic surgery is considered as acceptable by men as by woman. Currently about 20 percent of all cosmetic procedures are received by men, and every year that number grows. The reality is that our society rewards a more youthful look, and this affects both men and women.

MYTH: ONLY RICH PEOPLE ARE ABLE TO GET COSMETIC PROCEDURES.

REALITY: Once upon a time only the rich and famous were able to get plastic surgery, but those times have changed. Average, everyday people are getting cosmetic procedures. According to the American Society of Plastic Surgeons, two-thirds of people who undergo cosmetic procedures have an annual household income of less than $60,000. We are not concerned with your income level; rather we want to work within your budget to help you feel better about yourself and the way you look.

MYTH: ONLY VAIN PEOPLE GET PLASTIC SURGERY.

REALITY: Every person wants to look his or her best: How we look is closely connected to how we feel. People who are vain are totally obsessed with looking good at the exclusion of reality. Vanity means never looking good enough and having the desire to have more of everything. The desire to look your best and to have your outward appearance reflect how you feel inside is a natural aspiration. We find that most of our patients simply come in wanting to make cosmetic changes in order to feel better about themselves. Seeking plastic surgery is not about being vain, but rather about having the courage to stand up and do what is best for you. Getting surgery is a big step that will change your life. When you feel better about yourself you will see that you start living a fuller life.

MYTH: PEOPLE ARE NEVER HAPPY WITH THEIR COSMETIC PROCEDURE RESULTS.

REALITY: Yes, there are stories out there about plastic surgery disasters, but these are rare and often happen because people went to someone who wasn't skilled, trained, or even a real, bona fide surgeon. There are also those individuals who see how easy one change was and decide that they want more. This isn't dissatisfaction, but rather a desire to keep improving their look. Research at the Clevens Center for Facial Cosmetic Surgery has found that the majority of our patients are pleased with their results. Interestingly, our studies have shown that the only regret in over 80 percent of our patients is that they wish they had decided to have their procedure done sooner.

MYTH: COSMETIC INJECTIONS CAN REPLACE THE NEED FOR A FACELIFT.

REALITY: Although cosmetic fillers can do a lot to create a more youthful facial appearance and might be able to postpone the need for a facelift, they cannot replace the effects that a facelift will create. When there is significant loose skin and droopiness of the facial muscles, all of the fillers in the world will not be able create the transformation that a facelift can. If you are on the fence about a facelift, it is a great idea to try out fillers to see if these give you enough change to make you happy with the way you look. Stick with the fillers and non-surgical solutions so long as you are pleased. You will know when it is time to begin considering surgical alternatives.

MYTH: COSMETIC PROCEDURES DON'T NEED
CHECK-UPS AFTER THE PROCEDURE.

REALITY: Your procedure doesn't end once the surgery is over. A conscientious surgeon will want to work with you through the entire healing process and up to at least one year following surgery to make sure that you are happy and healthy. Plus, close follow up and the implementation of a coordinated skin care and maintenance plan help you keep your look fresh for as long as possible. Getting check-ups after your procedure will help to confirm that everything has gone according to plan and that you are healing properly. At The Clevens Center we want to ensure that we have exceeded your expectations.

MYTH: YOU HAVE TO HAVE GENERAL ANESTHESIA
WITH PLASTIC SURGERY.

REALITY: There are some procedures where general anesthesia may be recommended, but this isn't the case for every procedure. Many cosmetic surgeries can be done under different forms of sedation. This can include twilight sedation, local anesthetic, or even just a topical numbing agent. It is dependent on the procedure. Many procedures are now being performed in the comfort of the office or with light sedation. The goal is to ensure your safety at all times and to be certain that you are comfortable during your procedure.

THE CATALYST

a t Clevens Face and Body Specialists, we have seen many people from different walks of life come through our doors. These patients all have a unique reason for deciding plastic surgery is their next step, but they all have one thing in common: an event that served as a catalyst for taking action.

THIS MOMENT IS

FROM THINKING

It could be the shock of seeing a recent photo. It could be someone mistaking you for someone much older than you actually are, or it could be a significant birthday passing. But for everyone who decides to get plastic surgery, there is a catalyst moment.

You might have been thinking about it for a while and vacillating on whether it is right for you or if you are really ready. At some point there is an event that pushes you over the edge. This moment is when you shift from thinking to taking action.

That catalyst moment is important to remember. It will provide clues about what is important to you and why you are walking down this road to a better you.

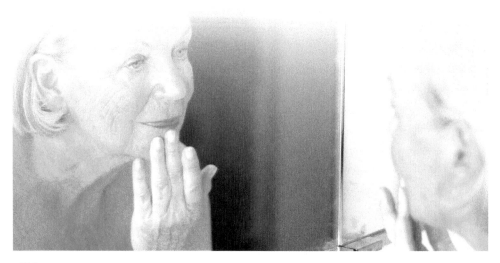

HOW DID THIS VISIT MAKE YOU FEEL?

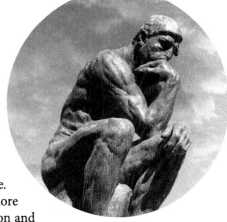

Congratulations! You have taken the first step on your journey to a successful facial procedure. Only six more steps! There is just one more item we want to discuss with you before we move on and that is to reflect on your first step.

Now that you have met with the staff and been to the clinic of your choice, we really want to encourage you to stop for a moment and check in with yourself about how you feel. How are you feeling about the process thus far? This is another important opportunity for you to use your journal and take notes of anything that comes up for you. After meeting with the professionals at your clinic, do you still feel comfortable? Were they friendly, cordial, helpful and understanding? Did you learn things from them? Do you know more now than before you came in? Do you believe that they will be able to help with your desires and expectations? Are you confident that you can move forward and actually do this? Are you now empowered with a stronger sense of who you are and what you want? Do you feel safe? That is, do you feel that you will be in good hands during this process that may change your life?

Most importantly, do you feel that you have been **heard**? Remember our quotation by Robert Frost? Did the medical team talk too much and make you feel that the conversations were one-sided with too much discussion about them? Do you feel like you were truly listened to and that you learned more about yourself through the process? Did they address all of your concerns about this very important decision? After all, this entire process is about you and they need to know your concerns. The principle objective is that your needs and your expectations are all brought to the forefront. The professionals need to have heard your concerns and fully understood and acknowledged them. You need to be heard and they need to understand.

At this point you should be feeling pretty excited and inspired. After all, you've been thinking about this for a long time now and you've finally made the move. You made the decision; the hardest part is over. You have started the momentum moving forward. Your surgery is getting closer, and soon you will have a new reality to your appearance.

Good for you! You have shown the courage and the strength to take this first step, and we take our hats off to you for a job well done. We totally understand that it hasn't been easy for you. We highly respect you and your decision.

PEOPLE IN THE KNOW
PERSONAL TESTIMONIALS

k eep in mind that even with all that you have been through by this stage, you are not alone. Over ten million Americans each year elect to undergo cosmetic surgery. Many people have gone before you and have experienced the very same emotions that you have. Others have felt all the fears, doubts, anxieties, excitement, joy, and uncertainties that you have gone through. To help you see how others have dealt with these same issues, here are what a few of our recent patients are saying about their experience of going to a plastic surgeon for the first time.

A recent Dr. Clevens patient is Naomi, a 44 year old office manager for a Fortune 500 Company. She experienced a lot of apprehension, confusion, and doubts before she took the first step towards plastic surgery.

Even just bringing myself to the clinic for the first time was a great challenge. I had done all of my homework. Hour after hour I would research the backgrounds of plastic surgeons – but to actually go to the clinic and talk to somebody about my issue was very difficult for me. When I finally did start going to clinics, I never felt right. I would have to wait for a considerable length of time, or I wouldn't feel very comfortable with the staff members. I even went to Los Angeles and consulted with some of the plastic surgeons of the stars. But what an experience that was. They made me feel like 'cattle' – get in and get out as fast as possible. When I heard about Dr. Clevens through a friend of mine here in Florida, I thought I'd give him a try. Again, as I said before, just getting into the center was a great challenge for me, but I made myself do it. My first visit was an eye-opener. I was impressed with the look of the office, and the staff was very friendly and accommodating. In my first visit I was surprised that I didn't meet with the surgeon, Dr. Clevens. I was expecting to, but the staff that I did meet with spoke to me like a real person – woman to woman – on my level. I felt comfortable and assured that I was doing the right thing. I was so impressed that I couldn't wait for my second visit and actually meet Dr. Clevens."

Remember, a journey of a thousand miles begins with the first step. You have taken this first step – you are now well on your way. Congratulations again! The next step? We will see you in the doctor's office, fully prepared, for your unique consultation with your facial plastic surgery specialist. ◼

YOUR **NOTES**

_____

_____

_____

_____

_____

_____

_____

_____

_____

_____

_____

_____

_____

_____

_____

_____

_____

_____

_____

_____

CHAPTER TWO
STEP TWO
THE SPECIALIST
ADVANTAGE

Your Consultation with the Facial
Plastic Surgery Specialist

OUR **FIRST MEETING**

t this point in your journey you will have already met with the facial cosmetic surgery staff of your choice and had your initial consultation about your unique concerns and what you want to have done. You have started your surgical journal and have begun to really look at your hopes, dreams, and fears surrounding your cosmetic procedure. The staff of professionals has helped to get you started and made you feel secure with the direction in which you are headed.

Trust forms the very foundation of the patient-physician relationship. Cosmetic surgery has become commercialized and heavily advertised. With this promotional fanfare, the importance of the patient-physician relationship has become lost. It is important to recognize that cosmetic surgery is a branch of medicine and, as such, merits a keen measure of seriousness and importance based upon a foundation of trust…trust that your doctor is ethical, skilled and up to date with the latest advances in medical and surgical care. Remember that your doctor is your advocate and he or she should have your best interests in mind at all times.

You are not buying a commodity that can be compared on the internet; you are hiring a surgeon to perform a job for you. Like an artist or a musician, you are relying upon the hands and expertise of your surgeon to perform for you upon your command and to create a surgical outcome that fulfills your aesthetic dreams and aspirations. This is not a skill that can be branded, boxed and sold on TV in an infomercial or packaged and resold on the internet. It is all about your trust in your surgeon and whether you feel confident in his hands.

The staff members at qualified facial cosmetic surgery centers are highly skilled and trained professionals who are experts in the art of listening. In our Center of Excellence, our staff members have been working and communicating together for many years. You should trust that the concerns that you have shared with them have been related to your surgeon with strict confidentiality and accuracy. As a result, you can be sure that if you do have questions or concerns you can speak with anyone in the office and they will be able to help you.

At Clevens Face and Body Specialists, our dedicated support team is here to educate and inform. They want to help you in any way they can, believing that education can help to relieve many of the most common uncertainties. With that being said, please ask questions. Ask as many questions as you want and don't feel afraid or embarrassed to do so. An educated patient is the best patient. Educate yourself about your journey and never forget that the professionals are available to help – every step of the way. They will always have your best interests foremost in mind.

No less important than qualifications, training, and experience is how a surgeon makes you feel. Take a moment to ask yourself how your prospective surgeon made you feel during your visit. Establishing a good rapport with the surgeon, or any doctor that you work with, is essential. In the cosmetic surgery arena, you will have a close relationship with your surgeon and his staff for some time prior to your surgery and for at least one year afterwards. It is important that you are comfortable communicating with him and his staff. All of these things come into play in what we consider the second step in this process: "The Specialist Advantage." You deserve an expert who has specialized in the field of plastic surgery that most closely matches your area of concern.

THE SPECIALIST
ADVANTAGE

etting The Specialist Advantage is when you and the surgeon get together one-on-one and talk about your needs and your expectations from your experience. After all, the facial cosmetic surgery experience is about YOU – the patient. It's about helping you determine what will make YOU happy. The venture is unique to each individual – there isn't a one size fits all "cookie-cutter" approach. Every patient brings to the table a unique set of concerns. The major goal of the surgeon and his or her staff is to transform your concerns into the appearance that you've always dreamed about.

It is not unusual for patients to want information on their doctor's credentials and experience before moving forward with that surgeon. This is important information to have and it is another part of The Specialist Advantage. All board-certified facial plastic surgeons (www.abfprs.org) have to go through many years of rigorous study, training, and examinations to get where they are. Remember to seek a surgeon who is a specialist, board certified in the area that you are concerned with. Getting the details of any surgeon's education, training background, certifications, safety record, and success rates should be an important part of your choosing whom you will work with for your plastic surgery procedure.

THE AESTHETIC
GAME PLAN

his consultation is about you, which means that your facial cosmetic surgeon and his or her staff will spend most of the time together talking about your concerns. Imagine your surgeon had a magic wand and could create the transformation of your dreams. What would those changes look like? This is your opportunity to share your dreams and hopes.

Although there may be some generally accepted principles of what we find attractive, beauty is truly within the eye of the beholder. Every individual is endowed with a unique appearance and style. In facial plastic surgery, professionals must respect and build upon your individuality to create a transformation that is uniquely your own and fits your vision of beauty. You should understand that true beauty comes from within, but sometimes you need a little help in finding that beauty within you. People are under a lot of pressure to fit into what society tells us we need to look like. This pressure can take its toll on your self-esteem. A good facial cosmetic surgery center will want to help you boost your self-confidence and acknowledge the beauty that you already have.

It is helpful to hear how long you've been feeling unsure about the way that you look and why you feel that now is the right time to consider changes to your appearance. Many surgeons will actually enjoy learning the reasons why these concerns have led you to their center. In your explanation, be clear, precise, and honest. Trust is paramount in any relationship. After all, your face is special and that's why it's the only specialty at our Center of Excellence that focuses on facial plastic surgery rather than plastic surgery in general.

During the consultation the surgeon will conduct a thorough examination of the topics that you have outlined. Through this process he or she will be able to assess what options might help you achieve your desired appearance: what can be done to change your facial structure, what needs to be done, and, perhaps most importantly, what should not be done. Together he will go over all of these opportunities and discuss your options in detail.

our facial plastic surgeon will use video imaging that can show you what you will look like after certain procedures have been completed. He or she will share exactly what will be done in surgery and display the corresponding predicted results. You should bring up any potential worries, questions or suggestions. This will help him or her to further visualize the exact results that you desire. In this phase of the process you are exploring all of the possibilities. Remember, at this point you are working on developing a partnership; honesty, sincerity, and trust are all essential keys to the successful outcome of your surgery. Above all, you deserve an expert who has specialized in the field of plastic surgery that most closely matches your area of concern.

Video imaging is an important teaching exercise where your surgeon and the staff are able to exchange ideas. Computerized preview imaging allows them to simulate changes, add procedures, delete procedures and modify procedures.

Going back to our example of the rhinoplasty and chin implant scenario mentioned in Chapter One, let's say you're interested in nasal reshaping and contouring (rhinoplasty). After a thorough evaluation, a chin implant is suggested. If this wasn't part of your game plan, you may not envision what the professionals see in their analysis. So, they can perform imaging of your likeness after rhinoplasty both with and without a chin implant. This allows you to see their vision and, most importantly, empowers you to make an informed decision about whether you prefer your new look with

OUR FACIAL PLASTIC SURGEON WILL USE VIDEO IMAGING THAT CAN SHOW YOU WHAT YOU WILL LOOK LIKE.

or without your chin enhanced. The key here is your satisfaction. The professionals may make suggestions based upon their experience, however, you are the final judge of what is best for you. Nevertheless, they are available to help you along the way.

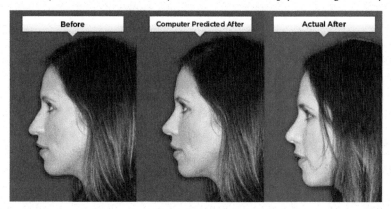

| Before | Computer Predicted After | Actual After |

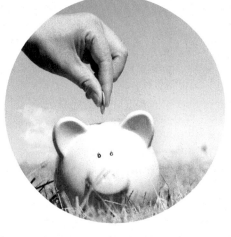

A WORD
ABOUT **COSTS**

nce you and your team have made a game plan and gone over all of the best options for your procedure, you will talk about the costs. Plastic surgery can be quite costly and the specific fees vary greatly depending on the details of what is being done. Together you will go over the basic costs and come up with a proposed financial investment. Your professionals will make every effort to detail all of your costs in advance of your procedure so there are no surprises or hidden costs.

Not all plastic surgeons charge the same. In our connected internet world, comparison shopping is easier than ever. Keep in mind that you are not purchasing a commodity such as a loaf of bread or a carton of milk. A facelift is not a facelift is not a facelift. There are lots of techniques, outcomes and certain risks.

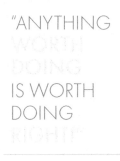

"ANYTHING
WORTH
DOING
IS WORTH
DOING
RIGHT!"

You have only one face and this may be the only opportunity in your life to have your facelift, rhinoplasty or eyelid lift properly performed. As my father used to say, "Anything worth doing is worth doing right!" Remember these words.

We encourage you to shop around, but your emphasis should be on trust, experience and skill, not price. Here is a word of warning: Be wary of any surgeon that is offering special 'offers' or 'discounts.' If it sounds too good to be true, then it probably is.

Deep down, we all know that's the case. Certain doctors are not scrupulous and make promises that they cannot or will not keep. Your face is far too important to risk by taking bargain deals. We guarantee that you will grow to regret your cosmetic surgery bargain.

e would also offer a word of caution against any doctor that is overly aggressive, tries to place pressure on you to get surgery, or who attempts to push you into getting unnecessary or unwanted procedures. This type of behavior is not only unprofessional but also deceitful. It is abhorrent to everything that facial plastic surgery is really about and to all of those dedicated professionals who work in our field.

"THE AT OUR CLINIC IS THAT YOU HAVE

The philosophy at Clevens Face and Body Specialists is that you have come here after serious thought. You have already invested enormous amounts of time to research and discussion. You have already looked at what is best for you. You have already started making decisions pertaining to your health and well-being. The qualifications, professionalism, and experience all direct your chosen facial plastic surgeon towards what is best for you and what is in your best interest. Ultimately, only you can determine what is in your best interest.

Your surgeon and his staff should appreciate the time that you have already put into this process. The goal of the surgeon is to listen to your concerns and lay out a surgical blueprint and care plan for you that is straightforward and direct. This is an acknowledgement of your experience and the realization that this is your face we are dealing with – and, in our practice, we take that very seriously.

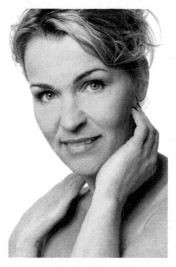

The goal of the surgeon is to listen to your concerns and lay out a surgical blueprint and care plan for you that is straightforward and direct."

THE
PRELIMINARY
TIMELINE

*a*t this point you have already been through a lot. You have met the professional staff and started the discussions with your surgeon. You have created a journal for your process, your expectations, and your questions. You have explored the details of your facial issues. You have talked about the pricing, potential concerns for the surgery, and how things will progress. Hopefully through this process, you have also created a comfortable rapport. Now it is time to talk about the preliminary timeline for your Aesthetic Game Plan.

> I SUGGEST TO ALL OF MY PATIENTS TO **USE THEIR JOURNAL** TO START WRITING DOWN **A LIST OF ALL THE THINGS THAT WILL NEED TO BE DONE BEFORE, DURING AND AFTER YOUR SURGERY.**

No doubt you have already started to put a game plan together. During this session with your surgeon and his or her staff, you will have gone over exactly what your surgery will entail, how much time off you might need from work, your pre-surgical preparations, the place where the surgery will take place and post-op preparations.

It is imperative that you are properly prepared and fully informed. As we have said before, an educated patient is the best patient. Educated patients know what to expect, anticipate what they'll need and become most pleased with their outcome. Thus, a good surgical team will want to educate you as thoroughly as possible. It is important that you feel comfortable, confident, and self-assured all the way through the process.

The following information serves to answer some of the more standard questions that tend to come up during The Specialist Advantage. Going through a cosmetic surgical procedure will change and affect your day-to-day life for some time. This information will further build on what you have already learned during The Knowledge Builder process.

TIME OFF WORK

O ne of the most common questions I am asked is, "How much time will I need to take off from work?" It might seem like time off from work should be the same for every patient, but in reality every patient heals differently. Some patients bounce back in no time at all. They cover up their spots, lumps and bumps with makeup and get right back into the swing of things. Others avidly guard their privacy and remain hidden until every last vestige of surgery has been resolved.

Based on my experience over the last twenty years as a facial plastic surgeon, I can accurately provide my patients with what I call "the three levels of healing." These 'levels' are specific to each individual procedure and tailored to each individual patient based on my knowledge of the patient and how I think he or she will fare in my best judgment.

THE FIRST LEVEL is when you, as a typical patient, are able to apply makeup
and look good to the point where most people won't recognize that you've had anything done. You may have some lingering lumps or bruises and perhaps a trace of surgery here and there. But, at this point, many patients return to work and resume their daily activities. For many procedures this may be a week or two.

THE SECOND LEVEL is what I call " the mother of the bride." This means that you
have an important event coming up, perhaps a wedding or a reunion, and you need to look terrific. At this stage of your recovery, you look great! No one will discern that you've had surgery and you have resumed all of your ordinary activities with no worries related to your healing process. By 6-8 weeks, most patients have achieved this level of recovery.

THE FINAL LEVEL of healing, for all procedures, is typically reached a full one
year after your procedure. It truly takes one year for the body to heal after a surgical procedure. It takes incisions one year to fully heal and there may be some subtle or episodic swelling, lumpiness or bumpiness that may take up to one year to fully resolve.

We recognize that cosmetic surgery is elective and that there are 'costs' related to your procedure beyond the surgical fees. There is the cost of lost time from work and play. It is important to be able to provide you with an estimate of time off that is as accurate as possible. It is important to us that you are pleased with your experience. A great many considerations, beyond merely the technical outcome of your procedure, factor into the definition of patient experience and satisfaction. If we do a great technical job and tell you that it will take three days to recover, but instead it takes three weeks, I guarantee that you will not be pleased. It is all about honesty and candor between the doctor and patient in creating expectations that are trustworthy.

PRE-SURGICAL **PREPARATION**

here is a lot that goes into pre-surgical preparations, but one of the most important parts of this process is the preparation that you make with your family and friends at home. For your surgery and recovery time you won't be as available as you usually are to your family. It is important that you make clear and concise plans for your absence in order to help your healing process.

What this really means is that you need to make arrangements for the redistribution of day-to-day tasks. This may include tasks at work and at home, and such daily tasks as housework, cooking, transportation for kids, routine phone calls, taking care of pets, watering plants, computer work, paying the bills and the like. No doubt, there are many people in your personal and professional life that depend on you and for these people you have probably been a major focal point of their lives. You have been the one that they go to when they need something, and any kind of absence whatsoever will be hard felt for these individuals.

We suggest that you use your journal to start writing down a list of all the things that will need to be done before your surgery, during your surgery, and afterwards.

This is just a simple list to help you get your things in order and to help make sure that you don't forget anything. Once you have your list completed you can start to talk to family and friends about what you will need during this process and who you will expect to take care of what. You can also write lists for the people who are going to help you with your day-to-day tasks as you recover. This list will serve as a guide for you and will always refresh your memory to help avoid confusion.

An interesting dilemma that many of my patients will share with me before surgery is "whom should I tell?" Do I tell my adult children that I am having a facelift? Will my mother be upset that I'm having my nose reshaped? What if my sister voices disapproval? These are all very common and interesting questions and each is as unique as the individual that poses the question or offers the answer. Many patients feel distressed by such questions from their friends and family.

The decision to proceed with appearance-based surgery is a very personal one that rests upon your own values and decision making and your own set of well-founded reasons for wishing to proceed with facial plastic surgery. This should be something that you are doing for yourself and not for someone else. You should not have to contend with the motives and influences of others once you have settled upon the course to recognize your dreams of achieving your desired look. We have found that those closest to you, who love you, who appreciate your desires and thought processes, will be most supportive of your decision to act upon your wishes.

SURGERY **LOCATION**

he location of your procedure is based on the nature of your procedure as well as your overall health and well-being. Many procedures are performed safely and comfortably within the privacy of your surgeon's own state-of-the-art clinic, while other procedures are more appropriately undertaken at a nearby ambulatory surgical center. This facility should be certified by the state and accredited by national credentialing organizations ensuring that it meets the highest standards of excellence and safety.

Often, an outpatient surgery facility is more convenient than a large hospital and is typically staffed with specialized doctors, nurses and assistants. Surgical center professionals work hard to make your experience as pleasant as possible and to provide a continuity of care. You will always see a friendly face that cares about you.

THE LOCATION OF YOUR PROCEDURE IS BASED ON THE NATURE OF YOUR PROCEDURE AS WELL AS YOUR OVERALL HEALTH AND WELL-BEING.

PAIN

everyone fears pain. This is a natural and evolutionarily adaptive response. However, it is interesting that the level of discomfort experienced after facial surgery is dramatically less than that experienced with other sorts of surgery. Facial surgery is considered much less uncomfortable than breast or body surgery and certainly much less painful than surgery upon a bone or joint, a hysterectomy, C-section or nearly any other sort of major surgery.

After facial, neck, eyelid and nasal surgery, studies have shown that many patients don't complain of pain at all. Instead, most patients report a sense of pressure or tightness. Although you may fear pain, pain is not a common aspect of facial surgery and should not be an obstacle to fulfilling your goals.

Despite our reassurance, though, we find that patients want to be told how much pain they will experience both during and after surgery. To address this, a good center for facial cosmetic surgery will have created an active community of current and former patients who are willing to share their experience with new and prospective patients. This is a valuable network that helps individuals better prepare for their procedure and manage their expectations around the time of their procedure.

If your procedure is performed under anesthesia, then you will feel no pain at all during your procedure. Although many fear anesthesia and ask to avoid it, modern anesthesia is exceedingly safe with the risk of a serious unfavorable occurrence falling in the 1 in 800,000-1,200,00 range, which means anesthesia is safely administered in greater than 99.99% of cases according to recent studies. Having said this, however, it is not uncommon for some patients to feel nausea or disorientation for a few hours after the administration of anesthesia. The first few days after your surgery may also be marred with discomfort. However, please keep in mind that many patients merely require nothing more than Tylenol to relieve the pain.

It is important to remember that every patient is different. Pain tolerance and pain control will be different for each individual, and we work hard to treat you as an individual. If your pain increases or persists, we can make prescription pain medication available.

RISK AND SAFETY FACTORS

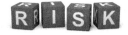

a s with any surgical procedure, there are certain risks and safety factors which must be taken into consideration. This information is intended for general education purposes only and should not be relied upon as a substitute for professional and/or medical advice.

Complications rarely arise, and these can have varying side effects, either short-term, long-term or both. Often the potential side effects are connected to the specifics of the cosmetic procedure that was performed or by the anesthesia itself. Greater than expected bruising, swelling and slow healing are a few of the more common complications.

Another possible complication is an unfavorable result. This means that despite the best efforts of your surgeon as well as your strict adherence to aftercare instructions, sometimes things just don't turn out the way we had all hoped. This does occur from time to time even in the best of hands. Most statistics show that this occurs in up to 10% of all cosmetic surgery cases, making it the most commonly encountered complication in plastic surgery. It may be the result of poor communication, unrealistic expectations or just the way the body heals.

THE BEST AND MOST EFFECTIVE WAY TO AVOID ANY RISKS OR COMPLICATIONS IS TO HAVE A THOROUGH AND COMPREHENSIVE PHYSICAL BEFORE UNDERGOING SURGERY.

However, there are several ways to keep surgical and anesthetic complications to a minimum. The best and most effective way to avoid any risks or complications is to have a thorough and comprehensive physical before undergoing surgery. This will help to ensure that your body can stand the rigors of anesthesia and surgery.

Any misinformation conveyed to the doctor performing the physical prior to the surgery may lead to serious ramifications during surgery (more on this in chapter three, pertaining to your health and well-being assessment).

ou can also avoid serious complications by following directions with your antibiotic medication. After surgery it is common to take prescribed antibiotics. A patient can become seriously ill if prescription medication is not taken properly. Antibiotics should always be taken until the medication is finished and not any sooner. Feeling better isn't a sign that your medication should be stopped. Antibiotics are prescribed for a certain length of time because research and experience shows that this duration is necessary.

Getting all of the pre-operative screening taken care of will also help to ensure your procedure will go smoothly, minimizing the risk of complications and unfavorable outcomes. The screening will vary depending on your health history and the surgical procedure that you will be getting. The screening could include blood tests, x-rays, heart studies such as an electrocardiogram (EKG) or stress test and any other tests deemed necessary for your health and well-being. These tests will help to confirm that there aren't any medical complications that could interfere with your anesthesia and surgery.

Slow healing can be caused by certain lifestyle choices. For example, smoking before or after surgery or frequent and long term exposure to the sun can cause problems. It is important to follow all of the directions that you are given post-op in order to have a complication-free recovery time.

Overall, complications arising from plastic surgery are quite rare. If you follow instructions and adhere to everything your surgical team tells you, both before and after the surgery, you will have a safe, worry-free and rewarding experience. Your professional team will follow you through your timeline every step of the way: They are dedicated to your health and well-being. This whole process is about you, and you can be assured that you are in good hands with them.

There are some more common complications and less common risks. Here are a few that you need to be aware of. Remember that knowledge is power and having this information will be important for you going forward.

HEMATOMA} A hematoma is bleeding underneath the skin that clots and can cause potential complications leading to more surgery. This is a rare issue and affects only 1-3% of people who get plastic surgery procedures. It is a more common risk in men than in women and in smokers than non-smokers. In smokers the risk may exceed 10% depending upon the type of surgery. Hematoma formation is more common in patients who continue blood thinners around the time of surgery against medical advice, who have high blood pressure or who are more active than instructed after surgery.

SEROMA } A seroma is like a hematoma, but instead of blood collecting under the skin, clear non-bloody fluid collects. It is most common in surgery where a lot of skin is lifted and fat is contoured or removed. This can often be prevented with proper wound drainage. It is a more common risk in patients whose activity level is too strenuous after surgery or who do not wear their compression dressings after surgery as instructed. Seroma formation is also more common in smokers.

NECROSIS } An uncommon complication, but a serious one, necrosis is when the skin tissue begins to die and fall away from the incision sites. This happens when there isn't sufficient blood supply and tends to be more prevalent in smokers.

NERVE DAMAGE } Any time the skin is cut there is a potential for nerve damage. Nerves may be stretched during plastic surgery procedures, but the problems come into play when major nerves are damaged. Nerve injury is a risk with all surgery and can be permanent. This could lead to permanent or temporary muscular weakness depending upon the type of nerve injured.

INFECTION } Uncommon in facial surgery but the severity of the infection can vary depending on the individual and the procedure. Infection isn't considered a major issue with cosmetic procedures because most individuals getting plastic surgery are considered healthy and the face has a strong blood supply that helps fight off infection. This risk is greater in smokers than in non-smokers.

HYPERTROPHIC SCARRING } This is when the scars from surgery are thick and red. Most often serious scarring is avoided because the surgeon strategically places the incisions in areas where they can be hidden. This risk is also greater in smokers.

NUMBNESS } Temporary numbness is very common following cosmetic procedures. People have rarely experienced permanent numbness at the incision site or surrounding areas.

BLEEDING } This is a very uncommon issue in facial surgery and in only one percent of cases is there bleeding that can cause serious issues or complications.

PTOSIS } Sagging or drooping can happen after several different facial cosmetic surgeries or even a Botox treatment. This is rare and with Botox will dissipate on its own within a few weeks time.

LOOKING OPERATED UPON OR OVERDONE } A good cosmetic procedure isn't going to be obvious. Good cosmetic surgery is going to help you look better, but what is more important is that it helps you to feel better about yourself. Selecting an experienced facial plastic surgery specialist should help you achieve a natural or rested appearance.

DO YOUR
RESEARCH

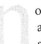o doubt you have already done research and put in-depth thought into what kind of surgeon you want to perform your procedure.

Part of that research is determining qualifications and experience. Just by the fact that we are talking, I am going to assume that you will be looking for my knowledge, expertise and experience in this field; and indeed you should be.

This is a given, for truly no one wants to be the subject of a poorly trained or inexperienced surgeon – especially when it comes to such important matters as your face. Your face is special and that's why, at Clevens Face and Body Specialists, it is our only specialty.

BE CONFIDENT
THAT YOUR FACIAL
PLASTIC SURGEON
CAN REALLY
HELP YOU.

Be certain that you select a specialist board certified by the American Board of Facial Plastic and Reconstructive Surgery (www.abfprs.org) to care for your facial aesthetic and reconstructive concerns.

You need to be confident that your facial plastic surgeon can really help you. This is a turning point. It is important to me that my patients feel secure in my professional background and credentials to perform your particular surgery and fulfill your needs. You need to know this information not only to feel confident but also to ensure that you are doing the right thing with the right doctor.

As much as you need to get to know your surgeon, your surgeon has to get to know you as well. In my practice, I have to determine whether or not you would be a good candidate for facial plastic surgery in the first place.

Many prospective patients come to me with unrealistic expectations and under misconceptions that plastic surgery is going to cure their depression, make them more socially acceptable, or guarantee wealth, health and happiness. I need to know whether or not your true motivations for plastic surgery are heartfelt, unfeigned and realistic.

"I have certain expectations of my clinic team's interactions with prospective patients."

Were you well received by them?

Did you feel comfortable?

Was your visit educational and informative?

How did you find the overall environment of the clinic?

Was your first visit really what you had expected?

Were you more self-assured about the possibilities or were you left with more questions than answers?

Do you feel like you were heard? That is to say, did you feel that my staff truly listened to you and your concerns?

Did you feel that they genuinely cared?

These are important patient-focused elements that are designed to improve patient experience and allow them to get the answers they need in order to become an informed and educated patient. After all, knowledge is power and the key to success in your facial plastic surgery journey.

Once you feel confident that your initial experience has been a good one, we can start to put a plan into place for how to best move forward. This is a template that we follow in my practice based upon my experience and your surgeon should follow a similar model.

BE CERTAIN THAT YOU SELECT A SPECIALIST BOARD CERTIFIED BY THE AMERICAN BOARD OF FACIAL PLASTIC AND RECONSTRUCTIVE SURGERY TO CARE FOR YOUR FACIAL AESTHETIC AND RECONSTRUCTIVE CONCERNS.

DR. CLEVENS

At this point you might be asking yourself, "But what about you, Dr. Clevens? Who are you? What are your credentials? What makes you stand out amongst the crowd of Plastic Surgeons and Facial Plastic Surgeons that could take care of my face?"

These are all great questions because you need to know about the person who is going to perform a delicate operation on something as important as your face. Let me take this opportunity to tell you about me. What follows is not boasting or self-promotion. It is a description of my experience and training and I challenge anyone to match it. I want you to feel confident that you are in good hands and that you have made the right decision should you decide to visit our Center of Excellence.

I am a well-trained medical doctor, specializing in cosmetic and reconstructive facial plastic surgery and MOHS skin cancer care. I received my Bachelor of Science degree, summa cum laude, from Yale University. After Yale, I completed eleven additional years of intensive training in medicine. This included earning my Medical Doctorate degree, magna cum laude, from Harvard Medical School and a Master's degree in health policy and management from the Harvard School of Public Health.

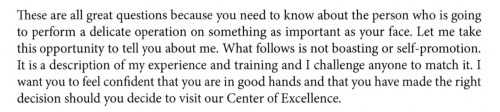

DR. CLEVENS **IS DOUBLE BOARD CERTIFIED** BY BOTH THE AMERICAN BOARD OF **FACIAL PLASTIC AND RECONSTRUCTIVE SURGERY** AND THE AMERICAN BOARD OF **OTOLARYNGOLOGY**

My postgraduate education entailed an Internship with the Department of General Surgery, Beth Israel Hospital, Harvard Medical School and Residency in the Department of Head and Neck Surgery at the University of Michigan where I was also appointed the Chief Resident in this department. I was awarded a prestigious Fellowship in Facial Plastic and Reconstructive Surgery at the University of Michigan.

I am double board certified by both the American Board of Facial Plastic and Reconstructive Surgery and the American Board of Otolaryngology – Head & Neck Surgery.

I was voted "One of America's Top Doctors," "Best of Brevard" by the readers of Florida Today and "One of America's Top Physicians" by the Consumers' Research Council of America and "The Reader's Choice Award in Plastic Surgery."

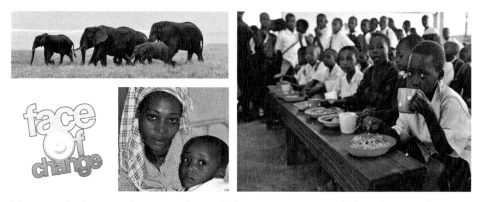

I have received various honors and awards during my career, including the Prize for Investigative Work, Columbia University College of Physicians and Surgeons and the Leon Reznick Memorial Prize for Excellence in Research at Harvard Medical School. I hold various professional affiliations, including the title of Past President of the Florida Society of Facial Plastic Surgeons, Fellowship in the American Academy of Facial Plastic and Reconstructive Surgery, Fellowship in the American College of Surgeons and Fellowship in the American Academy of Cosmetic Surgery.

Nearly twenty years ago I founded the Clevens Center for Facial Cosmetic Surgery, a nationally recognized Center of Excellence for facial plastic surgery in Melbourne, Merritt Island and Suntree, Florida. I am the Clinical Assistant Professor of Plastic Surgery at the University of Central Florida, College of Medicine. At the present time, I am the only practicing Board Certified Facial Plastic Surgeon between Stuart, St. Augustine and Orlando in Central Florida. We have recently renamed our center "The Clevens Face and Body Specialists" to reflect our bringing on board plastic surgeons with specific expertise in cosmetic and reconstructive surgery of the breast and body to complement my unique specialization in facial surgery. So, now our patients benefit from specialty care in each aesthetic region of the face, breast and body.

Beyond my medical background, I am also very proud to say that I am the president and founding partner of the charitable foundation Face of Change where we provide meals to the underprivileged both locally and abroad. In the last few years alone, through Face of Change, we have provided over half a million meals to needy children in our community. I frequently travel to Africa and other areas of the underdeveloped world, where I lead physicians on humanitarian missions to perform surgery and provide medical services to impoverished children. My African trips are profoundly moving experiences. It is some of the most rewarding and satisfying work that I do in my life.

In addition to being a doctor, I am also a husband and father. I have a beautiful loving wife, Dani, and two wonderful sons, Bernie and Max, who just call me Pops. We live with our dearly beloved dogs: a standard poodle named Lance, our toy poodle called Ginger, and our cherished chihuahua named Thor.

CHOOSING YOUR
SURGEON

W e want you to work with a surgeon that makes you feel secure and confident about your procedure. It is important that you find a doctor that is reputable and safe. Below are some warning signs that a surgeon may not be someone you should trust:

PRESSURE | A reputable surgeon should never pressure you into something that you don't want. Anytime you feel pressured or forced into procedures that you are not so sure about, you should walk away.

BAD MOUTHING COLLEAGUES | Among properly trained and well-qualified surgeons, there should be a level of collegiality and mutual respect that befits the medical profession. If your surgeon is drawing comparisons or slandering his or her colleagues, this should raise concerns.

IGNORING YOU | This whole process is about you. If your medical team isn't listening to you or not taking your interests into consideration they are not someone that you should be working with. Surgeons often fail to recognize that the process revolves around the patient, not themselves.

BARGAIN PRICES | Doctors might post special deals or promotions that they are featuring, but you should be wary of anyone that is offering their services well below what is considered the average price range.

SHORT CONSULTATION | Your visit with the surgeon should take as long as it needs to. They should be willing to answer all of your questions and take their time with you. If your potential surgeon seems to be rushed or unwilling to take the time that you need, he or she might not be the right doctor for you.

OVER PROMISING | It is important that you work with a realistic doctor. If your potential surgeon makes too many promises there is a very real chance that they might not be able to deliver on all of them. All this will do is lead to disappointment for you. If it sounds too good to be true, it probably is. We all know that good things don't often come easily. There are no shortcuts in life. As my father used to say, "Anything worth doing is worth doing right."

FINAL THOUGHTS
ON THE SPECIALIST
ADVANTAGE

We believe that it is important for you to know the background of your surgeon and his or her team. It is truly essential that you have as much information as possible. Remember, knowledge is power. Plus, by choosing a facial plastic surgery specialist you are entrusting him or her with your full confidence. It is important that you know just who this person is and who is going to be responsible for realizing your dreams for your appearance.

Now let's go back to you. It is extremely important from our point of view that you know just how you feel after talking to your chosen professionals in the consultation session. Do you feel better now than when you first came in? Do you feel more knowledgeable about what you want to have done? Have you been heard? That is, do you feel that they listened to you and have acknowledged your desires and needs? Do you feel respected, safe, connected, and confident? These are the questions you need to ask yourself as you prepare to move forward towards the next step of your journey.

You have now taken step two. Congratulations again! You know a little bit about the professional facial cosmetic surgery specialist and what he or she can do for you, and the professional knows a little bit about you. The next step? Let's go together, straight into step three: The Preparation and Reassurance Program (Your Health and Well-Being Assessment). ▪

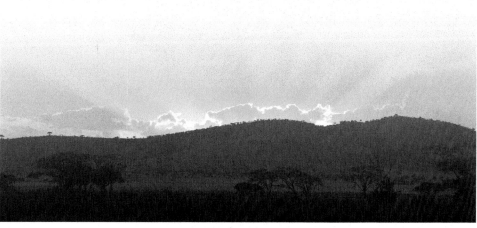

PEOPLE IN THE KNOW
PERSONAL TESTIMONIALS

Beth, a forty nine year old retail executive who traveled from Los Angeles for her surgery with me, had the following to say about her experience with us:

" *Dr. Clevens was truly amazing. I was expecting a rather cold, scientific person with a matter-of-fact personality. However, nothing could be further from the truth. Dr. Clevens approached me with a very warm and personable demeanor. What struck me the most was that he spoke to me and not at me. He put me at ease immediately, as if we were already mutual friends. He called me by my first name and made me feel important, as if I were the only one in the world that mattered to him. Dr. Clevens is confident in his experience. I was also really impressed by the fact that Dr. Clevens only works on faces and nothing else. That says something to me – a type of reassurance. I have a friend who had facial surgery done by a general doctor: She never felt right about the process and the results were very disappointing for her. I felt Dr. Clevens' expertise and knowledge was so impressive that when I left his office I had no doubt that I was with the right doctor. I was also very excited that I had actually found a person, after all my searching, that had genuinely listened to my concerns and actually acknowledged what I was saying. When I left the office after our meeting, I felt good, connected, respected, and safe. My first visit with him truly exceeded my expectations."*

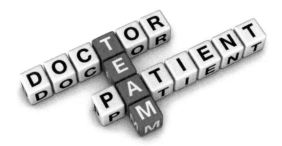

YOUR **NOTES**

_____

_____

_____

_____

_____

_____

_____

_____

_____

_____

_____

_____

_____

_____

_____

_____

_____

_____

_____

_____

CHAPTER THREE

STEP THREE
THE PREPARATION AND REASSURANCE PROGRAM

YOUR **HEALTH** AND **WELL-BEING**

his brings us to the third step in the process of making your facial plastic surgery a reality. We call this part of the journey "The Preparation and Reassurance Program." It is at this stage of the program that you, the patient, will start to make your own personal preparations for the surgery itself. Since you have decided to move forward with the procedure, you are now going through the process of putting the wheels in motion. You are taking the steps to make your decisions a reality.

At this point you will have done all your homework. You will have taken your time in pondering all the pros and cons. You will have had all of the necessary conversations with your friends, family, patient care coordinators, nurses, and your choice of surgeon. This is the point where you know exactly what you want and how you are going to get there.

For The Preparation and Reassurance Program, the process begins with a review of your personal health history. This will be done with your patient care coordinator, surgeon, and the anesthesiologist. All of these professionals will need to know if there are any diseases or disorders that you have had in the past or are dealing with currently. This is going to help them determine if there are any special issues that may need to be addressed before your procedure.

This information is intended for general education purposes only and should not be relied upon as a substitute for professional and/or medical advice.

YOUR PERSONAL
MEDICAL HISTORY

ny active or ongoing medical problems or disorders will be discussed at length. This is for your own health and safety. In order to ensure your health and well-being during the course of your procedure, it is important that you let your medical team know everything about your health history. To be certain that we have learned all that there is to know, your healthcare team will ask you. Indeed, it is common and at times frustrating that you will be faced with the same sorts of questions again and again. In medicine, we are trained to build this redundancy into the system to avoid medical errors. It is prudent for you and your care team to take a moment to write down all of your active and prior medical problems, prior surgical procedures, and current medications, including doses and when you take them. You will also want to mention any known allergies and personal or family history of difficulty with anesthesia or bleeding problems.

Some of the medical conditions that your medical team will want to know about are:

Heart problems
Vascular difficulties
Respiratory disorders
Easy bruisability or bleeding
Skin conditions
Allergies or Asthma
Digestive or Thyroid function issues
Neurological disorders
Diabetes
History of difficulty with anesthesia

Several of these medical issues require ongoing medication and medical management to deal with the symptoms. Some of these medications may interfere with anesthesia or the healing process. This is just another reason that you need to fully disclose your medical history to your surgical team. Never just stop taking medications. Your team of caregivers can usually find a way to work with you, but we have to know what we are dealing with first. Although, with some of the more serious medical issues, we might recommend that you not pursue cosmetic surgery at all.

UNHEALTHY
HABITS

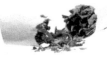

b ecause we are concerned with your overall health and not just your medical concerns, it is also important to discuss any past or present unhealthy habits or addictions to drugs, alcohol, or smoking. Your medical team will be able to give you some advice on how to deal with these addictions both before and after the surgery. Drugs, drinking, and smoking can all cause serious, life threatening complications during any medical procedure. It is imperative that you are open, honest, and up front around any addictions that you might be dealing with or have dealt with in the past.

If you are a smoker it is important that you stop smoking, at the very least, two weeks prior to your surgical procedure. Smoking can cause a series of both minor and major medical complications. Smoking can damage the incision sites from surgery.

CAN ALL CAUSE SERIOUS,

DURING ANY MEDICAL PROCEDURE.

This can lead to infection and poor healing. If infection isn't taken care of, or smoking continues during infection, this can lead to skin loss or necrosis, which is when live skin tissue begins to die and fall off. Smoking can also cause complications with anesthesia, pain relief, and the longevity of your surgical results. Smokers tend to bruise more than non-smokers and are more likely to encounter problems with bleeding.

Smoking damages skin. Smokers take longer to heal from surgery and the results of cosmetic procedures don't last as long in patients that continue to smoke after their procedure has been completed. Some facial plastic surgeons will advise a patient to quit smoking altogether due to the negative ramifications that smoking has on one's facial appearance and overall health.

If you are a smoker and have ever considered quitting, your facial procedure should serve as a great incentive to leave this nasty habit behind.

MEDICATIONS

t he professionals you are working with will also need to know what kind of medications you are currently taking. Remember, when it comes to plastic surgery every patient is unique and every surgical procedure is designed according to this uniqueness. The particular medications you may be taking need to be discussed before your operation.

This will ensure that any chronic medical condition you may have is under the right medical treatment and will put at rest any fears or uncertainties you may have about your medications. It will also further strengthen the rapport with your surgeon and build even further confidence in moving forward with your decisions.

Even nutritional supplements and over-the-counter drugs have the potential to have adverse effects on surgery. Anything that you are taking on a regular basis needs to be revealed. Aspirin and aspirin products, or any kind of cardiovascular medications, for example, should be avoided at least two weeks before and after surgery. This will

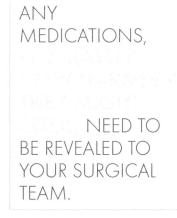

ANY MEDICATIONS, NEED TO BE REVEALED TO YOUR SURGICAL TEAM.

help to prevent any complications that may arise with the viscosity and constitution of the blood. Tylenol would be an excellent alternative here. Of course, as already stated, never stop taking medications without discussing it with your doctor and the medical team.

Any medications, no matter how harmless they might seem, need to be revealed to your surgical team. This will help avert unnecessary medical complications during or after your medical procedure.

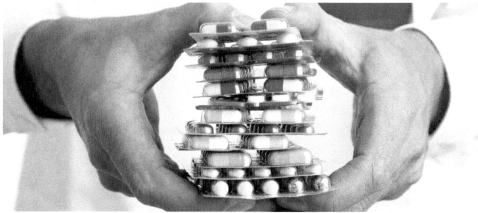

DIET AND WEIGHT

ou will also need to discuss your diet and any weight concerns you may have with your medical team. Your diet will give clear clues to your overall health and well-being. It is important that you are getting the best nutrients and vitamins before your procedure. This will help your health throughout the process.

Furthermore, your surgical team will need to know your weight gain/loss history. This might seem unimportant, but this information can help to determine whether or not complications could arise during the procedure.

For example, if you have experienced significant weight loss, either as a result of diet, prior surgery or health-related, we should know. A healthy, nutritional diet should be maintained in order to ensure a good, vibrant complexion, a solid sense of well-being, a speedier recovery and a longer lasting result of your new appearance. A healthy diet is important for being at your optimum health before your procedure. A healthy diet is a balanced diet. Enjoying a lot of fresh vegetables and fruits are important. Eating lean meats and complex carbohydrates, such as whole grains, will help to keep your body functioning at its optimum level. Avoid fatty meats, fried foods, sugars, and processed foods. It is also important to drink plenty of water while avoiding soft drinks and excessive caffeine.

Patients often come in to see us either after a significant weight loss or on the verge of a planned diet. What is most important with facial surgery is that your weight is relatively stable. Although facial appearance and facial surgery is far less influenced by weight gain or loss than body and breast surgery, we have found that the best results are achieved when you are within twenty pounds or so of your stable, baseline weight.

If you are about to launch on a diet to lose fifty pounds, I would suggest that you delay surgery until after you have lost your desired weight and maintained the loss for at least six months. By the same token, if you have just lost fifty pounds and are about to head off to your facial plastic surgeon for that makeover you've always dreamed of, I'd suggest you wait a few months to allow your weight to stabilize before you consent to surgery.

MENTAL HEALTH

our mental health is also of great importance to us as professionals and your support team. We will need to know if you have had any issues related to mental health, for this will assist in determining whether or not you are prepared for this rewarding process.

For example, if you suffer from depression, no amount of brilliant plastic surgery is going to help you to recover from this condition. If you are seeking plastic surgery as a means for dealing with your depression, this is the wrong reason. Your support team will want to be clear that if depression is something you are living with, you should not have false impressions regarding cosmetic surgery and what it can do for you going forward.

IF YOU **SUFFER FROM DEPRESSION, NO** AMOUNT OF BRILLIANT **PLASTIC SURGERY** IS **GOING TO HELP** YOU TO RECOVER FROM THAT CONDITION.

Plastic surgery helps you look as good as you possibly can. It also helps you look as good as you feel. Many patients feel great about their surgery and are grateful for their decision to address what bothers them about their appearance. Many patients find that facial plastic surgery helps them look and feel more youthful and competitive in the workplace environment. Better looking people earn more, gain more workplace promotions and are more persuasive. Plastic surgery can improve and boost your confidence both at work and in your personal life. However, it is important to realize that you are doing this for yourself. Plastic surgery will not fix a broken marriage, recoup a lost loved one, cure depression or change the world. You should feel comfort and gain confidence knowing we are helping you look the best that you can be – a look that matches how you feel.

On the other hand, it is not uncommon for patients to experience some sort of depression or melancholy after their procedure. This can be connected to many factors; one of these could be based on seeing the immediate results of bruises and swelling. It is natural to feel a bit down. After all, you spent all this money, underwent surgery and then you look in the mirror. Initially, you don't look as good as you were hoping. Feel comfort in the fact that everyone goes through this phase of melancholy, regret and wondering. With time, this will pass as the healing process progresses. If our staff knows that the blues is an issue for you, we will be better prepared to help you with any postoperative melancholy that might occur.

TIMING

Choosing the right time for your facial plastic surgery is also paramount for a successful outcome. When you are in the middle of major lifetime benchmarks, it is not the ideal time to undergo this type of endeavor. Marriage, divorce, separation, and the death of a loved one are just a few of the pivotal moments in life where your attention is directed elsewhere. Undergoing something as important as elective facial plastic surgery just might be a distraction that could wait for a more appropriate time when more attention and energy can be lent to this project.

> IS
> ABSOLUTELY
> PARAMOUNT
>
> WITH
> YOUR SURGERY.

Renowned author and motivator, Darren L. Johnson, once said, "I believe it is important for people to create a healthy mental environment in which to accomplish daily tasks." This could be taken one step further in saying that it is important for people to create a healthy mental environment in which to achieve successful facial plastic surgery. Getting into the right frame of mind is absolutely paramount in achieving a positive experience with your surgery.

Feeling positive and absolutely ready for your transformation is key for a successful surgical procedure and your mental well-being. You should feel excited about the adventure on which you are about to embark.

HONESTY

We have already discussed why it is imperative that you are totally honest and candid when revealing your health information to your healthcare professionals. The more we know about you and your concerns, the better we can all work together. You must not withhold any information; this could be very dangerous and could lead to grave surgical and anesthetic complications. No one wants to experience any surprises during the course of surgery. In helping us learn about you and your body, you will be helping yourself when it comes to enjoying a positive, pleasant, and rewarding experience.

After all that we have been through together, at this point we hope that you will feel comfortable sharing anything important with us. We are here for you, and as your medical team we want to be aware of anything that is going on in your life. Being open and honest with us will lead to your health, safety, and well-being.

THE PROCEDURE

O nce we have covered your personal health history, it is time to move towards the personal preparation stage of the process which involves the details of what we plan to do during your cosmetic procedure. We will discuss exactly what the surgery will entail and the steps that we will take to create the look you've always wanted. This will help you to visualize what is happening during the operation and educate you as to how we are going to reach the desired results. When referencing your education, we believe that we cannot emphasize enough how important it is for you to be knowledgeable. We feel confident that the more you learn, the more comfortable and happy you will be with us and the more satisfied and confident you will be with your choice in our clinic.

Do you remember when we walked you through the one-on-one consultation with your surgeon and his or her staff? You went over your concerns and charted out a course of action to take. Now it is time to review that plan again in your health team meeting. This is a perfect opportunity for you to refer to your journal and bring up any lingering questions or thoughts that you might have about the procedure. This meeting is a great time for you to mention any revisions or changes that you might prefer over what we have already agreed upon. Remember, in plastic surgery, every patient, every operation is unique: there are no cookie-cutter procedures. Your team members take your uniqueness and your personal concerns and make them theirs. This is about you and your well-being and nobody else's.

Your surgeon should use this time to go through the selected operation in detail. He or she will reiterate the approach and even provide you with illustrations and your own photo images. He or she will clarify the lines being made on your body and what these marks mean. Your surgeon will go over any incisions that are going to be made and discuss the functionality of each incision. This is also when the best process for healing any incisions will be conveyed.

We understand that for many people just the word incision can cause discomfort and worry. Let us assure you that the more information you have the better you will feel about the surgery. Talking through any concerns as they arise is going to make the whole process much smoother and easier for you. Recovery time not only depends on the particular procedure, but it also depends on the individual. Since each patient is unique, recovery times will often vary. In any case, preparation for at least some down time is absolutely necessary.

BELOW YOU WILL FIND A PRACTICAL LIST TO PREPARE
FOR YOUR SURGERY AND THE RECOVERY PERIOD THAT
IS ESSENTIAL.

INSTRUCTIONS ON YOUR **BEFORE** AND **AFTER CARE**

t might not seem to make sense to talk about post-procedural care before we even get into the details of the procedure, but before and after care are related. The things you do pre-surgery are going to help you post-surgery. And since this operation is about you, it will be you, and you alone, who will have the responsibility to "take care of business" before your operation.

Facial plastic surgery is a rebirth of sorts. You emerge with new looks and, we hope, a new outlook. Seize this as an opportunity to change your broader life and life's habits. Embrace a healthy diet, a healthy lifestyle and practice 'safe sun' with rejuvenating skin care.

> FACIAL PLASTIC
> SURGERY IS A
> REBIRTH OF SORTS.
> YOU EMERGE WITH
> NEW LOOKS
> AND, WE HOPE, A
> NEW OUTLOOK.
> SEIZE THIS AS AN
> OPPORTUNITY TO
> CHANGE YOUR
> BROADER LIFE AND
> LIFE'S HABITS.

This is an important stage because anything you forget to do prior to the operation will be much more difficult to accomplish following the operation. We suggest you get your affairs in order before the surgery.

The extent to which you need to prepare will depend on the complexities of the surgery and the amount of recovery time you require.

Logically, a simple operation that entails just a few days of recovery will not call for the same amount of preparation that it would take for a full, comprehensive face lift.

PRE-PROCEDURAL CARE
(ONE TO TWO WEEKS PRIOR TO SURGERY)

TAKE CARE OF YOURSELF FIRST

Your care is the most important element. Your good health and well-being is essential before you can take care of anybody else. You have to make sure that you are taking care of your own body through proper diet and exercise. You will want to make sure that you are eating foods that are giving you all of the nutrition that your body requires. Being in good shape for the operation can be very beneficial.

If you are taking medications, you will need to ensure that all of your prescriptions are up to date and that you have an adequate supply around the time of surgery. At this point your surgeon should have a clear understanding of any medications that you are regularly taking. If you and your doctor have made arrangements for you to stop or start medications, then this is the time when that will happen.

If you are traveling for your surgery or you will be staying away from home, remember to have an adequate supply of your regular medications with you. I recently operated on a patient who traveled from the Midwestern United States to our center in Central Florida who felt that it was not necessary to bring any of his medications with him for his surgery. Although your surgeon is usually able to reconstruct a patient's medication list and help obtain needed doses from the local pharmacy, this creates the potential for confusion and mistakes. It is always best to travel with your medications, whether you are going on vacation or traveling to have facial plastic surgery.

In general, your doctor will ask you to avoid certain over the counter medications like aspirin, ibuprofen, and other anti-inflammatory medications. These can increase bleeding and are not conducive to satisfactory healing after any surgical procedure. He or she will let you know when it is safe to resume these medications after your surgery.

During this time you might also need to stop taking any nutrition supplements, teas, and herbs. This is something that may have already been discussed during your consultation appointments. Keep in mind, these supplements could also cause complications and should be avoided until your are given permission. Some homeopathic remedies, nutritional supplements, vitamins and minerals can interact with anesthesia, impair healing and predispose you to bruising, bleeding and swelling.

Furthermore, any cosmetics or skin care products that you use should be used sparingly. This involves cleansers and other harsh products that you might apply to your face. Most make-up and basic soaps should not be an issue. But it is important to avoid anything that could cause a rash or allergic reaction. This is not the time to test out a new make-up product or try a new face cream.

Finally, if you smoke, it would be ideal if you could refrain from smoking as much as you can for at least two weeks prior to the surgery. It goes without saying that smoking is truly detrimental to good health. We all know that. Even smokers know it. However, regarding plastic surgery, smoking not only affects the blood supply to the skin, but it may cause increased bleeding, slow wound healing, and generate other issues. It may also be a contributing factor in how the surgery itself is performed. For example, the length of incisions, the placement of incisions, or both, may have to be modified due to this habit.

TAKING CARE OF BUSINESS

a s far as taking care of your affairs at work, there are many things that you could do to make your absence from work seamless and less worrisome. You should plan your dates off for surgery. Since cosmetic surgery is usually elective in nature, you can comfortably plan a time for your procedure that works well with your work schedule and personal obligations.

Your exit from work and play will be eased if the right people know when you won't be available. Friends and helpful colleagues will also keep tabs on what you need to do at the workplace after your period of absence. Likewise, your return to work and play will be eased by proper advanced planning. Maintaining an honest, sincere rapport with your superiors at work, plastic surgery or no plastic surgery, is always a good thing.

FRIENDS AND FAMILY

riends are always good to notify when going in for surgery for many different reasons. One of the reasons is similar to what occurs in the workplace regarding rumors. If your friends know of your surgery, then they will not wonder where you are or why they haven't seen you for a while. Knowing what you will be doing will quell the rumor mills. Friends won't be concerned that you are ignoring them or that something is wrong with the relationship. Besides, if they know you're in the hospital, or if you are just at home getting bed rest, they just might take the opportunity to pop on by and pay you a visit. If this is a worrisome thought, just kindly inform them that you would not appreciate any surprise visits during the process – no problem – no worries. True friends will truly understand.

Informing your friends will also help in preventing a mountain of emails, voicemails, text messages, or other forms of correspondence from building up and then requiring subsequent responses. Plus, friends are always good to have around, just in case you need them to help out, run an errand, give a ride to your child, or just be an ear for you to talk to. After all, that's what friends are for.

Family, however, takes on a completely different dimension when it comes time for a plastic surgery procedure. With family come the required obligations of fulfilling one's duties. For example, if you know you are going to be out for a lengthy period of time, or an undetermined period of time, it is best to face these obligations with energetic intensity; otherwise, there may be some unpleasant consequences that follow.

Make sure that all of your bills, including utilities, are updated and paid. If your financial affairs are not in order, your cable company will not understand your need for bed rest and your family might be left in a frenzied quandary with no internet, telephone, or television connection --absolute necessities in this modern day and age.

Transportation must be arranged, not only for you to go to and from the place of your operation, but also for your children or loved ones that depend on you for rides to and from their places of work, school, recreation and the like. Housework, chores, and domestic duties all must be addressed if you are to find your place of residence properly intact upon your return. Pets especially need special care and cannot be neglected. Children are still going to need to eat every day and the dishes will still need to be washed.

If you haven't made prior arrangements for all of your daily chores it can become very overwhelming and stressful. Post-surgery you need to be resting and healing, not trying to put out fires at work or unload the dishwasher. Addressing these issues ahead of time is going to allow the wheels of your daily routine to keep moving, even if you aren't the one at the helm. This is important; it will give you a nice, uninterrupted healing time frame.

HERE IS A SHORT CHECKLIST OF THINGS FOR YOU TO CONSIDER GETTING SET UP AHEAD OF YOUR PROCEDURE. BY DOING THESE TASKS AHEAD OF TIME YOU WILL HAVE LESS TO WORRY ABOUT WHEN YOU NEED TO HAVE YOUR ENERGY FOCUSED ON RECOVERY.

Prepare and freeze at least a week's worth of meals. Even if you have someone bringing you food or willing to take care of meals it is a good idea to have something ready just in case. Things happen and a care provider might not be able to meet all of their commitments to you. It is better to have something that you can easily heat up than have to worry about what you are going to eat when you should be resting.

Stock your refrigerator with food that is tasty and easy to chew after surgery. We have found that patients often enjoy a soft diet after their surgery. So, consider nutritious foods such as eggs, yogurt, cottage cheese, fruit, bread – whatever you like that doesn't require too much effort to chew and digest.

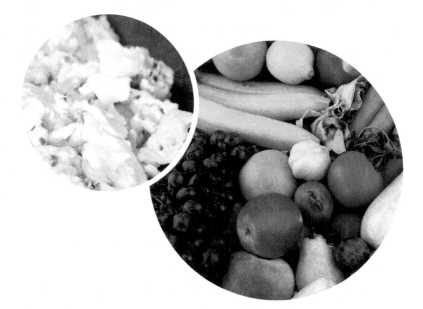

Be certain to have plenty of healthy drinks at home. Most patients do better with fluid other than water such as sports drinks (Gatorade or Powerade) and nutritious beverages (Enrich, Ensure, ideally with protein to encourage healing and with fiber to maintain regularity). Many patients take advantage of smoothies, protein drinks and other healthful liquids.

Eight glasses of water per day is mandatory. Increasing protein to one-and-one-half to two grams per kilogram of body weight is also important.

This is not a time to diet or lose weight. Your body requires a well-balanced diet with sufficient caloric intake to heal properly in order to have a good result from your procedure.

When packing for your surgery, remember to bring clothes that you don't have to pull over your head. Button-up shirts are going to be much easier for you to deal with when your face has just had surgery. Loose fitting clothes that are made of soft and natural materials are the best options.

Get any prescription medications ahead of time. It is better to have these medications already waiting for you at home, rather than trying to get your prescription after surgery. This will also help you to avoid any discomfort waiting to get your painkiller from the pharmacy.

Clean your house before your procedure. Coming home to a freshly cleaned house is going to help you relax and will prevent you from feeling the need to clean when you should be resting. Plus, a clean house means a house that has less germs and this can help your healing.

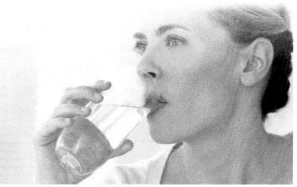

POST-PROCEDURAL CARE
(ONE TO TWO WEEKS AFTER SURGERY)

U pon returning home after surgery, there are many things that you must be aware of in order to ease your transition back to normalcy. In reference to your operation, you will still be feeling the effects of the anesthesia and other medications, so you will definitely have to take it easy for at least the first couple of days back.

Be careful about making sudden movements during this time. Medications will still be in your system and you might be feeling lightheaded or dizzy. For the first few days after your procedure, rest is the only thing that you should be concerned with. Other activities should be avoided in order to mitigate negative ramifications and even possible injury.

Some of the activities that you need to avoid during the first few days post-op would be things like:

> Driving an automobile
> Operating heavy machinery
> Lifting heavy items
> Leaning forward or bending over
> Participating in sports
> Strenuous exercise or sports
> Making any important decisions

As far as your wound care is concerned, you should not change dressings until your follow-up appointment, which will take place in your doctor's office.

You should always keep your dressings dry. Most often dressings will be changed in the clinic anywhere between the first 24 – 48 hours after the cosmetic procedure.

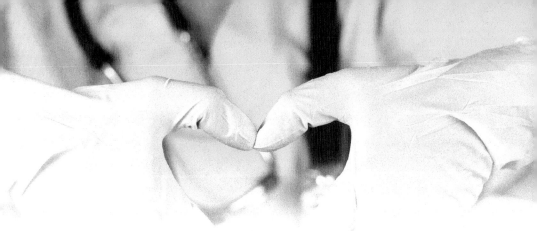

During this time and for the first week following your procedure, it will be important for you to try to sleep with your head somewhat elevated. The best way to do this is to get more pillows under your head or use a traveling pillow to keep yourself upright. This isn't always the most comfortable way to sleep, but it is important to do so for the first few days after surgery to minimize swelling and to promote healing. We have found that many patients sleep most comfortably in a recliner rather than a bed when first returning home after surgery.

At times during your recovery process you might feel overwhelmed so please keep in mind that someone should be available 24 hours per day to address your concerns. Although in our practice, my staff and I are with you all the way and available 24 hours per day, 7 days per week 365 days per year, it is important that you have someone at the bedside with you. We will help guide you through the steps weeks before the operation and we will still be there for a long time to come after the operation.

> RECOVERY PROCESS YOU
>
> OVERWHELMED,
>
> SOMEONE SHOULD BE AVAILABLE 24 HRS PER DAY.
>
> ALL THE WAY AND ARE AVAILABLE 24 HRS A DAY,

We believe that follow-ups are the major focal point for all successful operations. We are very concerned about your health and well being and monitor the healing process to the point of full, satisfactory recovery.

Upon your return to home after your surgery, it is time to take a few days off to allow the recovery process to kick in and do its job.

Now is the time to wallow in the well-deserved luxury of letting others pamper you for at least a few days. Float on the feeling that all is taken care of – all is good.

THE PATIENT CONCIERGE

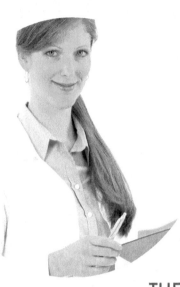

THE PATIENT CONCIERGE IS RESPONSIBLE FOR ALL OF THE DETAILS OF YOUR FACIAL PLASTIC SURGERY EXPERIENCE, **FROM THE FIRST CONSULTATION ALL THE WAY THROUGH TO YOUR COMPLETE RECOVERY** AND BEYOND.

he Patient Concierge is something unique to our cosmetic surgery center. Just as the concierge at a fine hotel ensures your comfortable stay, our patient concierge ushers you through your cosmetic surgery experience setting your mind at ease and tending to every last detail of your care. Having such a professional available is key to the healing process.

The Patient Concierge is an expert trained in the care of the facial cosmetic surgery patient. Our concierge is trained to make our patients feel good about themselves, to help them get well-prepared for their before and after surgery obligations and serves as a resource for comforting reassurance.

The Patient Concierge is responsible for coordinating all of the details of your facial plastic surgery experience, from the first consultation all the way through to your complete recovery and beyond.

The Patient Concierge tends to your needs, lifting some of the worries about managing your surgery: everything from coordinating transportation services for you, to helping with pre-operative obligations, to arranging nursing services at the post-operative stage. No request is too big or too small. Patient Concierges will handle any of the pre-operative quirks discussed above, such as making sure your pet gets what it needs, to the setting up of your home for proper post-operative care.

They work for your comfort, your safety, and for your peace of mind. At Clevens Face and Body Specialists, our patients meet frequently with our patient care concierges to help ease any apprehensions that you may have. A dedicated Patient Concierge can take care of all your needs, and it will be done discreetly and in total confidence.

FINALIZE YOUR
FINANCIAL INVESTMENT

nlike other branches of medicine, finances are integral to decision making in plastic surgery. Because cosmetic surgery is generally not covered by insurance, we must broach the subject of expense and financial obligations. With the surgical plan having been charted, finally we have reached the stage where we all must ensure that the proper legal and financial obligations are met. Although they are simply formalities, they must be addressed at this point before moving forward to the surgical experience itself. The consent forms must be properly completed and thoroughly reviewed; the form of payment must be established and submitted. Don't be reluctant to discuss the financial component of your cosmetic surgery. It is part of the process and it is important that you understand what is and is not included in your price quotation.

CONSENT FORMS

here are a variety of different consent forms depending on the type of procedure that you will be getting. Some are to provide written verification that your statements pertaining to your health are honest and true to the best of your knowledge; others are to provide personal permission to perform the surgery discussed and explained in our consultations. Apart from obtaining legal permission for your operation and evidence of your understanding and agreement to the procedures to be performed, there are forms to advise your family, forms that provide information pertaining to certain medications to avoid, forms to fill out if you smoke, forms for anesthesia application and forms to verify your understanding of pre- and post-operative instructions for your specific operation.

The process of obtaining informed consent is really an opportunity for both our office and our patients. The consent represents a chance for you to review the surgical plan, to clarify your expectations, to have your questions and concerns addressed and to fill in any blanks in your educational process. All of these forms are a necessity and may sound quite intimidating. However, the seasoned plastic surgery staff is available at all times to help you through this mundane, yet very important and necessary process.

FORM OF PAYMENT

INVEST IN YOU!

he form of payment must also be addressed at this point. Although many reconstructive surgeries are covered by plans offered by insurance institutions, most aesthetic or cosmetic surgical procedures are not covered by insurance companies. A good plastic surgery team is highly trained in providing you information on what can and cannot be covered for your particular case. It is customary with cosmetic surgery that all fees are paid in full in advance of your planned procedure. Because surgical schedules are busy and your surgeon has obligated his schedule and his staff to your procedure, it is common to expect payment in full one week to one month prior to surgery. It is further important to recognize that a significant portion of that payment may be non-refundable. Be certain to clarify the financial policies prior to submitting payment. The costs of your cosmetic procedure, including all the necessary services connected to it, are discussed in detail in Step One and are then modified in Step Two for any changes. Upon mutual agreement, the cost is then paid through various forms of payment.

Most centers are happy to accept your payment by cash, personal check, or credit card. It is certainly a great way to earn miles on your favored affinity card. If you are looking for financing for your cosmetic procedure there are several financial service institutions that your surgeon and his staff can recommend for you to look at for covering your costs. Keep in mind that most reputable centers for facial cosmetic surgery look upon the financial costs of your facial plastic surgery more as an investment as opposed to any type of procurement. Our philosophy is that your surgery is a wise investment in yourself, both for your future health and well-being.

PEOPLE IN THE KNOW
PERSONAL TESTIMONIALS

Patient Katie, a 44 year old golf professional, was more than pleased with her experience.

" *I have never had a doctor, not to mention a surgeon, call me personally and ask how I was after a procedure. This was something special. Dr. Clevens made me feel that I was important. He was genuinely concerned about my welfare.*"

Juan, a 29 year old rhinoplasty patient who had traveled from South America to have his nose re-done, had a very pleasant experience with the post-operative process.

" *Well, on the day of the surgery, I felt safe and confident in Dr. Clevens' skills. I felt very secure because Dr. Clevens and his staff gave me a great feeling of self-assuredness – confirming that this was really what I wanted to do. They all comforted me – I felt absolutely no pain whatsoever. And to top it off, Dr. Clevens came and visited me the very next day after I had returned home – on a Saturday! I felt honored that he would do this for me.*"

Now that all of the 'before surgery processes' have been addressed, let's move forward towards step four: The Tailor Made Surgical Experience. Onwards and upwards. Let's do it! ▪

YOUR **NOTES**

_____

_____

_____

_____

_____

_____

_____

_____

_____

_____

_____

_____

_____

_____

_____

_____

_____

_____

_____

_____

YOUR **NOTES**

CHAPTER FOUR
STEP FOUR
THE TAILORED
SURGICAL
EXPERIENCE

THE **DAY** OF YOUR **SURGERY**

he fourth step in the process of making your facial plastic surgery a reality is what we call the "The Tailored Surgical Experience." The day of the actual surgery has finally arrived. This is the moment when all of your preparations and hard work are finally coming to fruition. Reality is here; this is your big day. You will probably be experiencing some butterflies, but this is normal. After all, you don't do something like this every day. Nevertheless, you should take a deep breath and relax, knowing that you are in the hands of the best professionals in the business. They will take over from here. Remember, you have done your research. The team you have confidently chosen for your surgery is extremely well trained and experienced. They will make sure that you are comfortable, safe, and secure. You now know exactly what you want and the results you are going to attain. Embrace the moment and enjoy the experience.

Rest assured that although this is a unique experience for you, this is something that the professionals do every single day. The best way to gain expertise and proficiency is to do the same thing over and over, day after day. Although this may be your first facelift, be certain that this is not your surgeon's first experience. They achieve excellence through detailed processes and checklists day after day. Although I may have performed a thousand facelifts, each and every day I embrace the fact that this may be the first time for my patient and, as such, it is a very special day in their lives.

There are several steps to this phase, and each one has its own importance. Let's go through each of these points one by one so that you can be fully prepared when this exciting moment comes into your life. But before we jump into the details of the day, we need to back up a step to when The Tailored Surgical Experience really starts, and that is the night before the big day.

THE **NIGHT** BEFORE YOUR SURGERY

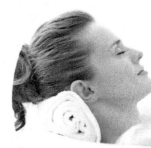

I n some ways your surgical process started two weeks before your actual appointment date. For those who smoke, you would have ideally abstained from smoking for at least two weeks prior to this day. The negative ramifications have been dealt with at length in Chapter Three. Furthermore, those who are under medication will be clear on which medications should be stopped and which should be continued. Having said this, however, regular medications should only be taken with a small sip of water the morning of your surgery subject to our specific instructions tailored to your unique set of medical conditions. Ideally, your stomach should be empty for at least 6-8 hours before your procedure and the surgical center staff will instruct you clearly on this matter. This will help your anesthesia go more smoothly on your special day.

The night before your surgery we recommend that you relax and be with friends and family. Being with the ones you love the night before a medical procedure can help to alleviate stress and lessen anxiety. You can also use this time to go over last minute family plans for your period of absence. Domestic chores and obligations that you usually take care of (and are usually taken for granted) should be thoroughly discussed and evenly distributed for equal responsibility. Who feeds the dog? Who takes out the trash? Who pays the upcoming cable bill?

Writing all these instructions down and giving copies to everyone concerned might be a good idea. Some patients have gone as far as placing their lists on their kitchen bulletin boards or even on a communal blackboard in order to make sure that everyone who needs to see the list has clear access to it and it won't get lost. This is also a good time to finalize plans. Your transportation to and from your surgery should be confirmed, along with all the details you have arranged with your 24-hour support person. Anything left out here could present inconveniences later on.

If you haven't already done so, now is a good time to pack your bag. You might only be gone for one day, but if you are expecting an extended time away, you will want to make sure that you have packed everything you will need for your comfort. Even a day's stay in the ambulatory clinic will require some indispensable things. Make sure that all your necessary paperwork is in order and included on your list.

Your personal identification, prescription medications, favorite bedclothes and your inseparable teddy bear, Saint Raphael's medal or whatever makes you comfortable should top off the lineup.

The last and most important thing that you need to do the night before your cosmetic procedure is take some time for you. Take a deep breath, relax, and find some peace with yourself. A nice calming hot bath or shower can do wonders for your peace of mind. This could also be a great opportunity to use some anti-bacterial soap or other surgical solution. Your surgeon will let you know what might be recommended for pre-surgery preparation. We also encourage you to remove all fingernail and toenail polish as well. This doesn't have to be stressful. Make this process a calm, soothing preparation for the adventure that you will be going on in the morning.

ARRIVAL AND CHECK-IN

a s you prepare to go to the surgical facility, you will want to make sure that you are dressed appropriately. That is to say, you are not going off to some gala affair or ballroom celebration. There is no need to try to dress to impress or make some kind of fashion statement. Save these outfits for more appropriate occasions.

For your cosmetic procedure you should be wearing loose-fitting clothes, and all jewelry should be left securely at home.

It would be best to not wear any of the following:

> Make-up
> Perfume
> Hairspray
> Contact lenses
> False eyelashes
> Artificial nails
> Dentures

Just come as yourself. Nothing else is needed or necessary. In fact, such things mentioned above could impede the surgical process.

Good, reputable ambulatory surgical centers are accredited. This means that they are state-of-the-art facilities that have been certified by the American Association for Accreditation of Ambulatory Surgical Facilities (AAAASF), The Accreditation Association for Ambulatory Healthcare (AAAHC) or The Joint Commission on the Accreditation of Healthcare Organizations (JCAHO).

These are the organizations responsible for setting the industry standards for best processes, supplies, equipment, staffing and physicians. You can trust that you are in the best center with the most qualified staff that meets or exceeds the most stringent standards for outpatient care.

YOU CAN **TRUST** THAT YOU ARE IN **THE BEST CENTER** WITH **THE BEST STAFF** THAT MEETS OR **EXCEEDS THE MOST STRINGENT PATIENT CARE.**

Upon arrival at the operation facility, you will enter the reception area where the surgical nurse will greet you. This person will be with you throughout your entire stay at the facility. His or her major function will be to make sure that you feel comfortable, safe, and self assured, with total confidentiality.

Before anything else, the staff on hand will need you to verify your address, contact numbers, consent forms, and they will make sure that you address any other necessary paperwork at the front desk. From there your surgical nurse will escort you into the change room. If you have any friends or family members with you, they can accompany you up to this point; however, they will be asked to stay behind when it comes time for you to move into the next stage of the procedure. In this suite you will change into a surgical gown, slippers and any other necessary gear for the surgery.

Now comes the time for you to meet with the anesthesiologist and then connect with your surgeon for the final pre-operative meeting.

THE **ANESTHESIOLOGIST**

our board certified anesthesiologist will talk to you first, principally to review your health history and go over the details of your previous meeting. He or she will also determine the kind of anesthesia that will be used and also will determine the constitution and strength of the chosen anesthetic.

To be most effective, the anesthesiologist will need to take into consideration such information as your age, body weight, body fat percentage, and your medical history. You will want to be fully honest and candid as no one is here to pass judgment.

The information provided will be imperative for the anesthesiologist to make the right choices for your surgical procedure. Remember, there should be no surprises on the operating table. Your safety is paramount.

The anesthesiologist is also going to ask questions pertaining to the last time you ate or drank. You should have been fasting for at least 6-8 hours prior to surgery, most typically from at least midnight the night prior to your procedure. This ensures that your stomach is empty during surgery and anesthesia. If you do have something in your stomach while anesthesia is administered, your risk of vomiting is increased and this can create complications during your procedure as well as uncomfortable nausea as you recover.

Therefore, it is important that you follow the surgical center's instructions and that you not eat or drink before your procedure unless otherwise specifically advised.

SIDE EFFECTS **ARE RARE** AND WITH THE **CONTINUING ADVANCES** IN MODERN MEDICINE, GENERAL ANESTHESIA HAS BECOME **REMARKABLY SAFE**.

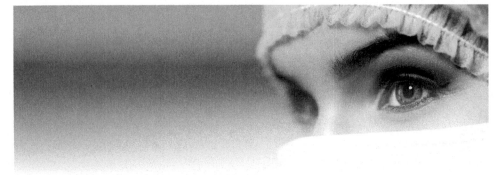

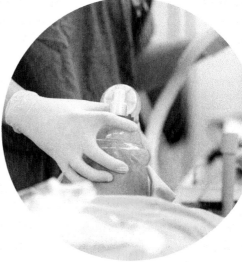

ou will want to mention to your anesthesiologist if you or any member of your family has experienced complications with anesthesia. This is also a time to list any medications and supplements you have continued to take. Some medications could have an adverse effect with anesthesia and may cause problems during the surgery.

The anesthesiologist is concerned with your maximum safety and wants everything to go smoothly and pefectly during the operation. No surprises!

Board certified anesthesiologists are fully qualified to perform their job dutifully and with the most distinguished of expertise. Anesthesiologists are full-fledged medical doctors (MDs) that are required to study and practice medicine for years before taking on full responsibility in the operating theater.

YOU CAN **TRUST** THAT YOU ARE IN **THE BEST CENTER** WITH **THE BEST STAFF** THAT MEETS OR **EXCEEDS THE MOST STRINGENT PATIENT CARE.**

However, their studies do not stop after medical school or residency, for the very nature of the constantly changing and evolving field of anesthesiology and pain management demands a lifetime of continuing education. The application of the proper anesthesia and the method in which it is applied is a craft that requires knowledge and expertise.

The anesthesiologist determines the type of application after your consultation in the facility. He or she will decide and confer with you about using a local, regional, conscious, or general anesthesia.

This information is intended for general education purposes only and should not be relied upon as a substitute for professional and/or medical advice.

TYPES OF **ANESTHESIA**

Local Anesthesia - This form of anesthesia involves the numbing of a specific area of your body and that specific area only. Most people have experienced local anesthesia. This is the type of anesthesia most commonly used by dentists or if you have ever had stitches. Numbing medicine is injected into the area that is being treated. Chances are you didn't feel the work being done, but you were fully awake, alert and you probably felt the medicine being injected to numb the area. Topical anesthetic creams can be applied before the injection of local anesthesia to 'deaden' the area before the shot of numbing medicine.

This type of anesthesia is common for minor cosmetic procedures or simple skin excisions for moles or small skin lesions. The benefit of this type of anesthesia is that it is simple and straightforward. There are very few risks, but it is not ideal for more involved or longer lasting procedures.

Regional Anesthesia - This type of anesthesia is also referred to as a nerve block. It covers a larger area of the body than a local anesthesia. An entire limb or the lower half of the body can be numbed using this anesthesia. Most often this form of anesthesia is used for women in childbirth and is more commonly known as an epidural or spinal epidural. As with the local anesthesia, a patient under a regional anesthesia can remain conscious during the procedure. Most often when it comes to facial plastic surgery, a regional anesthesia is applied for procedures like facial liposuction, lip augmentation, lip reduction, or a browlift.

Conscious Sedation - This type of anesthesia is more commonly referred to as "Twilight Sedation." This type of anesthesia is one of the favorites among surgeons due to its general safety and quick recovery time. It is often combined with a local anesthetic to further minimize discomfort. Under conscious sedation you feel relaxed, but remain awake during the procedure. Often, with deeper levels of sedation you are asleep throughout the majority of the surgery, but you can be easily awakened and you are breathing on your own.

Twilight sedation is most commonly administered through an intravenous line (IV). This form of anesthesia is frequently used for facial plastic surgery and is common for operations such as a necklift, blepharoplasty, skin resurfacing and many other common facial plastic surgery procedures.

General Anesthesia - This is the type of anesthesia where you are "asleep" for your procedure. Under this form of anesthesia you are totally unconscious and will not be able to recall anything that took place during your surgery. Under this form of sedation, the anesthesiologist places a breathing tube once you have fallen asleep. Once intubated, the breathing tube is used to maintain sufficient protection for the airway passages and the anesthetic allows for relaxation over a prolonged period of time. The anesthetic is relatively easy to induce and can be administered quite rapidly through the inhalation of gas or with an intravenous line. Side effects are rare and with the continuing advances in modern medicine, general anesthesia has become remarkably safe. The incidence of nausea and vomiting, once common with general anesthesia, has become very uncommon with facial surgery owing to the advances in anesthesia medicines and the introduction of strong medicines that successfully prevent post-operative nausea and vomiting.

At Clevens Face and Body Specialists, our anesthesiologists practice with the utmost knowledge and skill. With over 20 years of experience in the field, I have had more than enough time to survey my options of anesthesiologists and I always opt for the best in the business.

DURING YOUR OPERATION, OUR ANESTHESIOLOGIST WILL **CONTINUALLY MONITOR** AND **ASSESS YOUR VITAL FUNCTIONS** SUCH AS **BREATHING, HEART RATE, BODY TEMPERATURE, AND BLOOD PRESSURE.**

They are responsible for the condition of your sedation before, during, and after your surgery. Throughout the whole process they will stay in communication with me as your surgeon and any other medical practitioners. During your operation, our anesthesiologist will continually monitor and assess your vital functions such as breathing, heart rate, body temperature, and blood pressure.

As you can see from the information provided above, there are risks with the application of any form of anesthesia. Each application has its own distinct complications, reactions, and benefits. All precautions will be taken to minimize the potential dangers inherent in any anesthetic and ensure maximum safety with a successful outcome.

FINAL MEETING WITH THE SURGEON

fter having your very important and necessary check with the anesthesiologist, you will then meet with your surgeon. You already know each other from your first consultation and you should be comfortable with one another (see Chapter Two, The Specialist Advantage).

This pre-operative meeting will be somewhat brief, but important as these few minutes together will serve to touch base and go over some last minute details.

EVEN THOUGH **YOU MIGHT BE OUT OF YOUR COMFORT ZONE** YOUR SURGEON IS IN HIS ELEMENT AND WILL TRY TO MAKE YOU **FEEL AS COMFORTABLE AS POSSIBLE.**

You will also address any final questions or issues you may have pertaining to your cosmetic procedure.

He or she will want you to feel comfortable, relaxed, and good about yourself. If you are nervous, he or she will offer reassurances.

Being nervous is normal. Surgery is something that you do not do every day, and the surgeon understands that.

Even though you might be out of your comfort zone, your surgeon is in his element and will try to make you feel as comfortable as possible.

Our anesthesiologists are the best in the field. Indeed you can be fully and absolutely confident that you are in good hands with us every step of the way.

he great rapport you have established with your surgeon in previous meetings will carry forward. Together you will go over our planned procedure and touch upon a few details highlighted in your photo images.

The surgeon will then take the surgical pen and draw the landmarks on your face which will chart the course of the surgery. With a series of lines, dots, and arcs, he or she will quickly, yet with the greatest precision, mark the path for the necessary surgical incisions. Yes, you will look a bit like a road map after this process, but the operating room isn't far away.

THE SURGEON WILL **TAKE THE SURGICAL PEN AND DRAW** THE LANDMARKS ON YOUR FACE WHICH WILL CHART **THE COURSE OF THE SURGERY.**

At this point the surgical nurse will escort you into the operating theater itself for *"Your Tailored Surgical Experience."*

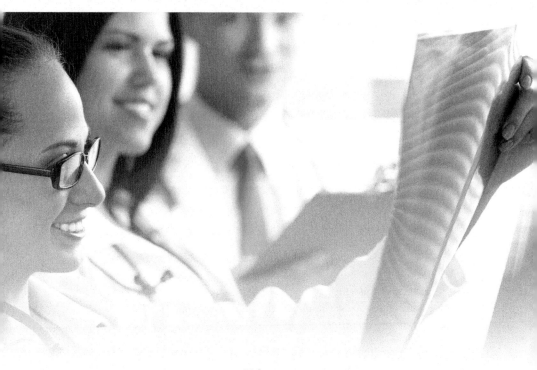

YOUR **AESTHETIC** JOURNEY BEGINS

s you enter the operating suite, you may be somewhat taken aback by all the people in the operating theater. The reason there are so many people is because the key components of your surgical team are all there: the anesthesia personnel, your surgical team and seasoned surgical care nurses. You really should not feel alarmed; all of these people are here for your best interest and safety. Every one of them is highly educated, licensed, and experienced. Each of them has a specific professional function, and each of them is working in a different and distinct professional field.

For example, the management nurse is responsible for taking care of the operating room materials. In order to hold this position, several years of training in the field of operating room management are required. The management nurse is also responsible for making sure all the materials needed for your surgery are readily at hand and are already in the room for us to use if needed. This includes items like sterilized surgical instruments, wound dressings, towels, and the like.

Without the hard work and dedication of the management nurse we would have to scramble every time an instrument or dressing was needed. Because of what he or she does, we are able to move forward with your procedure knowing that everything we need is already there and ready for us to use. A well-run operating room is like a symphony. There are many moving parts and lots of activity, but it should all come together flawlessly.

There will also be a registered operating room nurse who is responsible for overseeing all of the necessary operating equipment that is pertinent to your specific operation. This nurse is responsible for ensuring that all of the surgical machines that will be used are up and running in perfect working order. The operating room nurse runs tests on all of the equipment before the surgery starts in order to confirm that everything is running as it should be and won't cause any issues during the process.

Always present with me in my operating room will be the registered nurse or surgical assistant that works with me and with our patients in the office. She is a member of the American Society of Plastic Surgical Nursing (ASPSN) or the Organization of Facial Plastic Surgery Assistants (OFPSA). She has been working in surgery for nearly two decades and is certified and licensed to work in the plastic surgery and nursing professions. She is extremely efficient in what she does, which is rendering invaluable assistance to me in every aspect of the operation.

Of course, the anesthesiologist will also be present. When you first come into the operating theater, he or she will be going over all of the last minute details of the medication administration for your operation, as well as checking the machines. It might seem like there are a lot of us in the room, but you can trust that our operating suite is filled with highly educated and trained people with enough experience and laudable achievement to fill up anybody's Who's Who Book on Facial Plastic Surgery. No better hands are ready to serve you. It is now time to step up to our operating table; it's time to get to work..

THE OPERATION BEGINS

s you step up to the comfortable padded operating table and trust your face to the specialists, you will first notice a beehive of activity going on around you. As you lie on the table, the surgical nurse will take you by the hand and squeeze it as a reminder that we are all here to support you. As mentioned before, everyone in the operating room has his or her own specific function to perform. The surgical nurse is there to give you ongoing support.

All this bustling activity will probably be the last thing that you notice before the anesthesiologist connects you with the medications that will alter your consciousness. The medications that are used work with lightning-fast speed. As you drift off into the silent space of medically induced sleep, the bustle of the operating room will fade out around you.

As your awareness fades out of the room we get to work doing what we do best. No matter what procedure you have come in for, you can trust that we will take care of you with the highest level of skill and mastery. If you want to know more details about the specific procedure that is happening while you sleep, the following is information on the most common facial procedures. If you don't see your procedure here, more information is provided in Chapter Eight or at your own center for facial cosmetic surgery.

THE MOST COMMON FACIAL PROCEDURES

he following is information on the six most common cosmetic facial procedures that are performed. In the last chapter of this book (Chapter Eight - A Patient's Guide to the Most Common Facial Plastic Procedures), there will be more detailed information on what is frequently seen at centers for facial cosmetic surgery. In the meantime, since we are currently discussing the operation process for your personal transformation, here is what you might expect from the more customary procedures.

RHINOPLASTY

hinoplasty is the medical term for a nose job. This is one of the most common plastic surgery procedures that take place. The procedure works to improve the size, proportion, and overall appearance of your nose. Changing the nose can completely change the look of the face because it is such a prominent feature. Nose surgery can not only correct the size and shape, but also repair any internal structural damage that may impair your breathing and sinus function.

More than half a million people every year seek nasal surgery. When your nose isn't in symmetry with the rest of your face this is one of the most noticeable issues that you can have. Changes to the nose can be both dramatic and subtle; but no matter what, changing your nose will improve your overall look. It is important to consider the shape and appearance of your nose within the context of your overall facial features, facial shape and ethnic background. Your nose must fit with your overall look.

Don't be surprised if you think that you need nose surgery, but we suggest a chin adjustment either as an alternative to nasal surgery or in addition to nasal contouring. Often a weak chin can make the nose seem larger than it really is. Sometimes making a simple change to the chin can make the nose look to be in a more appropriate proportion.

During a rhinoplasty procedure there are two possible types of incisions that can be made. One of these is referred to as a closed procedure whereby the incisions are hidden inside of the nose and the surgery is done with small instruments from these incision sites.

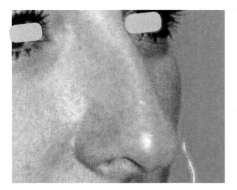   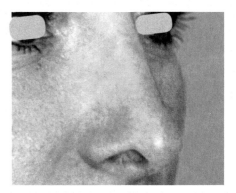

The other process is called an open procedure. During an open procedure the incisions are made around the nose and often, across the columella, which is the strip of tissue that separates the two nostrils. This is a more predictable and precise approach that allows for more access to the underlying structure of the nose.

With either type of procedure the tissue is then gently raised off of the structure of the nose. This allows us greater access to make the corrections needed. Once the tissue is out of the way we are able to reshape the bone and cartilage of your nasal structure. Occasionally, this means that we need to use cartilage from other areas of your body as a graft. If the septum, the piece of cartilage in the middle of your nose, is damaged, this is also when that area would be corrected.

Following all of the structural corrections the soft tissue is then replaced, or re-draped over your nasal structure, and any incisions are surgically closed. Depending on the work that has been done, excess tissue may need to be removed. This could also be dependent on the specifics of the surgery. Any external incisions are then sewn up along the natural lines of your face in order to keep them hidden.

Most likely splints, tubes, and other supports will be used to help keep the new nose in place for the night following the procedure. It is important that you follow all of the instructions that we have given you about post-op care. This will help your healing time to be quick and your pain levels to be manageable.

Swelling and bruising is common, but should subside in a few weeks time, but it will take up to a year for your new nose to fully finish the healing process and settle on your face. As you recover you will need to keep your head elevated. This helps proper drainage. You will need to avoid any activity that could put pressure on your face or cause damage to your nose.

EYELID SURGERY

yelid surgery is medically referred to as a blepharoplasty. In this procedure the eyelids are surgically adjusted to create a more youthful and rejuvenated look. An eyelid surgery can take place on the lower eyelids, the upper eyelids, or both depending on what your specific face needs might be.

You eyes reveal a lot about you. It is through the eyes that people are able to pick out your emotions and feelings. If your eyes look puffy, tired, or saggy this can convey emotions that do not convey how you really feel.

Some of the issues that an eyelid surgery can help are things like:

▶ **Removing the fatty deposits** that can accumulate in the upper eyelid. These deposits can look like puffy eyes and can't be helped with cosmetics.

▶ **Tightening up the loose or sagging skin** that starts to develop around the eyes. This loose skin can change the natural contour of the upper eyelid and can often cause the vision to be impaired.

▶ **Removal of the excess skin and wrinkles** that can develop around the lower eyelid.

▶ **Removal of under-eye bags that can develop.** These are actually fatty deposits that need to be removed and occasionally will require excess skin to also be removed.

▶ **Correction of lower eyelid drooping.** This drooping can often expose the bottom of the eye, which is a serious issue.

During the procedure any incision lines will be made in the upper eyelid crease where the upper eyelid folds upon itself as it opens. This will keep the incision lines hidden in the structure of your eye. The place where the incisions take place will mainly depend on what is being corrected with your eyes. Regardless, these small incisions allow your surgeon to reposition fat deposits, tighten the muscles, and remove any excess tissue if necessary.

∨ BEFORE; Actual Patient Eyelid Lift

∨ AFTER; Actual Patient Eyelid Lift

With the lower eyelid, incisions are often made inside the lower eyelid itself. From this area the fat can be removed or repositioned, the muscles can be tightened, and any excess tissue can be tightened as well.

Once the procedure has been completed the incisions are closed with either removable or absorbable sutures. There will be a certain amount of swelling and bruising that happens around the surgery site. Most often this will subside after a few days. Icing the area will help to keep the swelling to stay down and can help to speed up the recovery process.

Eyelid surgery is virtually painless and recovery is typically quick. After a week or two the area will be smoother and the surrounding areas will look more alert and youthful.

FACELIFT

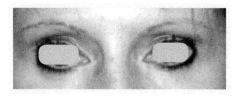

there isn't a specific age that is considered the right or most appropriate age for a facelift. The right time for a facelift is more about the look of your face than the chronological age. Many people are seeking facelifts at earlier ages than ever before. And the younger you get the procedure, the more subtle the changes will be and the longer your lift will last. Facelift creates the most dramatic and long lasting changes to the overall look of your face.

There are many types of facelift including the S-lift, Weekend Necklift, Direct Necklift, SMAS lift, deep plane lift and so forth. At this juncture, the point is to broadly consider facelift surgery as a procedure that rejuvenates the lower two thirds of the face and neck and not to get caught up in the particulars of each variation. The truth is that just as every face is unique, every facelift procedure should be tailor made to suit the individual patient's set of concerns.

The technical term for a facelift is a rhytidectomy and it is used to improve the visible signs of aging in both the neck and the face.

A facelift can help with the following issues:

> ▶ Facial sagging
> ▶ Creases below the lower eyelid
> ▶ Creases along the nose to the mouth edges
> ▶ Adjusting fat that has fallen or shifted
> ▶ Correcting loss of muscle tone
> ▶ Smoothing jowls
> ▶ Removing loose skin from under the chin & jaw line

It is common for people who are undergoing a facelift to have several other procedures done at the same time. Most often a browlift, eyelid surgery or even a nose job is combined with this procedure. It is also common to have facial implants, fat transfer, and skin resurfacing procedures done at the same time as a facelift.

The location of the incisions will vary depending on the specifics of your procedure. The most traditional facelift procedure uses an incision along the hairline around the temples. This incision will continue around the ear and often ends at the base of the scalp. Once the skin is loose, the fat can be sculpted, contoured or removed. After that, the tissue is repositioned and the deeper layers of the face and the muscles are lifted and tightened.

Once the reshaping is completed, the skin is re-draped over the face and any excess skin is trimmed away. If needed, an additional incision could be made at this point under the chin to further tighten the face. Sutures are made along the incision to close the wounds.

If the main focus of the procedure is on skin and fat under the chin, this might require a neck lift. For this procedure the incision is often made at the ear lobe and wraps around the ear to the base of the scalp. Since all of the incisions are made in the hairline and around the ears, they are unnoticeable after the healing process is complete. Any scarring will completely blend in with the natural shape and lines of the face.

There will be swelling and bruising after the procedure is completed, but after a few days this will slowly start to diminish. There is much that is required for the healing process from a facelift. Nevertheless, if you follow our post-op directions, you will be able to see the changes within a few days and will be able to return to normal activities within a few weeks.

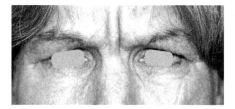 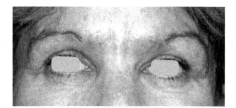

BROWLIFT

browlift is also referred to as a forehead lift. The procedure will lessen the creases that have developed on your forehead. These wrinkles are high up on the bridge of the nose and are often called frown lines. A brow lift will reposition the brow shifting the wrinkles and repositioning a sagging brow.

Many people start to show signs of aging on the brow before any other area of the face. Wrinkles on the brow can make it look like you are worried all of the time. How you normally wear your hair and how you feel about the creases in your forehead will determine how the brow lift will be done.

Most often a brow lift is done as an endoscopic procedure. In an endoscopic procedure, small incisions are made in the hairline and special surgical elements are used to make the cosmetic corrections. Because the incisions are so small in the hairline, once healing is completed the scars will not be visible.

The endoscopic procedure is preferred, when possible, because it has a quicker recovery time and it is generally less invasive. Once the procedure is done, the incisions are closed with removable or absorbable sutures.

There will be a certain amount of bruising and swelling after the procedure and this will last for several days. After a few weeks of healing and recovery the changes will be noticeable and you can resume normal activities. The effects of this procedure are permanent.

These are some of the more common procedures that we work with. Even with all of this information it is important to remember that each surgery is unique because each person is unique. Although the information provided is true about most of the surgical procedures, this information isn't true 100 percent of the time. Your center for facial cosmetic surgery will treat your operation as an individual procedure keeping your needs in mind.

SKIN RESURFACING

here are several different forms of skin resurfacing that can be used to treat wrinkles and discoloration of the facial skin. There are techniques that use a variety of lasers, amplified light, chemicals and mechanical forms of resurfacing such as dermabrasion and microdermabrasion. Each of these processes is applied to the top layers of skin to diminish blemishes and lines. Resurfacing will leave the skin looking smoother and younger because it takes off the damaged top layers of the skin. This system is one of the easiest ways to improve the appearance of the skin.

The following are skin issues that can be improved with using the chemical peel:

▶ Acne scars
▶ Acne
▶ Fine lines & fine wrinkles
▶ Freckles
▶ Irregular pigmentation
▶ Rough skin
▶ Scars
▶ Sun damage

Each of these techniques – laser refinishing, chemical peel, and dermabrasion – varies in strength and they can be adjusted depending on your specific needs. Your facial plastic surgery team will work with you to determine the technique that you need to make changes to your skin. Light resurfacing removes just the outer layer of skin and the process will provide a light exfoliation. Alpha hydroxy and beta hydroxy acids are common agents used in a mild chemical peel. The treatment can be repeated weekly for up to six weeks in order to get the results that you want. The light chemical peel is not going to remove deep wrinkles, dark spotting, or scarring.

The process is done by a nurse or aesthetician and is most often done without the need of anesthetic. To begin, your face will be cleaned and then the chemical solution will be brushed onto your skin. There can be a mild stinging sensation while the chemical goes to work. The chemical peel is then washed off.

Deeper peels and lasers treat the dermal layers of the skin and stimulate refinishing and remodeling of the skin that is long lasting. Typically performed as a single treatment rather than in a series, advanced laser techniques greatly improve even deep wrinkles, dark spots and scarring. Laser skin resurfacing is often performed at the same time as certain surgical procedures such as facelift, eyelid blepharoplasty and browlift.

ONCE THE **PROCEDURE** IS COMPLETE

W hen the last adjustments have been made and the final sutures have been placed on my work, the anesthesiologist will start to dial down on the medication he or she has been using to keep you asleep. At this point you will slowly and gradually awaken to the world that you had left behind so quickly. You will soon become lucid and be able to communicate, although you will be experiencing some new and strange sensations on your face.

The surgical nurse or nurse assistants will place you on a blanketed gurney and carefully roll you into the recovery room. Congratulations! The operation is over – you did it. From this point the recovery process has begun. Depending on your particular surgery and its estimated recovery time, there are a few things that could happen at this point.

One potential option is that after a couple of hours of observation you will be taken home by a designated driver. Another option is that you might be taken to one of our several recovery suites to stay for an extended length of time. Whatever the case, immediately after surgery and anesthesia wearing off, you will be in no condition to do any activity whatsoever. This is where all of the planning that you have done ahead of time comes into play. Since you have already made the arrangements necessary, now all you need to do is take care of yourself.

Being in the recovery room can be uncomfortable and strange, as the anesthesia is still wearing off. I am always amazed at how many people find the adventure much less of an ordeal than anticipated, especially those patients who undergo facial plastic surgery for the first time.

Facing the unknown and the untried is always filled with anxiety and anticipation. However, we have mentioned previously, most patients at centers for facial cosmetic surgery find the experience to be unexpectedly gentle and caring.

PEOPLE IN THE KNOW
PERSONAL TESTIMONIALS

Anne's makeover entailed a facelift, eye lift, and full face laser skin resurfacing:

" On the day of the surgery, I noticed that the nurses were all in a good mood. They were smiling and laughing… I wasn't nervous at all. There's something in smiles that is reassuring and relieving. I figured, if the people that are taking care of me are happy and content, then I should be, too. Shannon, the Surgical Nurse, came in and sat next to me. She held my hand and rubbed my back. She assured me that everything was going to be alright. Now that right there was tranquilizing in itself. Oh, and when Dr. Clevens came in, that just did it! Dr. Clevens has a way of calming you. He made me feel very relaxed. No wonder he got such high ratings all throughout my internet search. With all the other surgeons I looked at, Dr. Clevens was the only one that had perfect stars from all the patients that responded to survey questions about bedside manners. There were no complaints – not one. Knowing I was in such good care, I had no worries at all."

Anne went on to talk about her expectation of pain, but lack of it. "It was truly amazing, but I felt no pain. I almost felt like something was wrong because I wasn't hurting. Well, yeah, I was a little sleepy and groggy for the first couple of days, but after that I started feeling like Suzy again."

Lance, a travel industry executive, who underwent an endoscopic browlift and upper eyelid lift, also had a very positive experience in the operating room. She wrote:

" On the day of my procedure, I did sense quite a bit of anxiety; however, once I got to the facility, all of the staff really gave me a lot of assurance. I then felt really comfortable going into the O.R. During recovery I also felt comfortable. The staff continued to watch me carefully and they were all easily accessible. They were always very polite and professional."

lthough the patients listed experienced minimal pain during and immediately after their surgeries, this is certainly not to say that facial plastic surgery pain is nonexistent. In fact, all surgery bears a certain amount of discomfort, swelling, bruising, and puffiness to some degree. All recovery times will depend on the specific surgery and the individual. Many factors are involved in the recovery process, all of which will be discussed at length in the following chapter, "Chapter Five – Step Five - The Nurturing Process."

The average plastic surgery facelift operation will last anywhere from two to four hours. All other plastic surgery operations and procedures range anywhere from 15 minutes to several hours, depending on the surgical process involved. The recovery time can be especially long and what you do, or don't do, during this recovery time can truly make or break the actual surgery itself. This is why centers for facial cosmetic surgery pay special attention to the recovery process and emphasize its crucial importance. In fact, some centers have entire clinics dedicated to the process generally called centers for post procedural care.' More on this aspect in the next chapter.

THE TEAM MEMBERS ASK QUESTIONS TO GET A CLEAR IDEA OF WHAT THEY CAN BEST DO TO HELP YOU MOVE FORWARD AND GET STARTED ON YOUR ROAD TO RECOVERY.

Although you might still be feeling a little woozy from the process, the surgeon will want to know how you feel after the surgery is complete. Are you lucid or still groggy from the anesthesia? Do you feel like yourself yet? If you are experiencing pain, how much pain, and at what level of intensity? Just how intense is the natural feeling of swelling and puffiness? Do you feel nauseous? Do you have a headache? Can the staff get you anything? What would you like? Are you ready to go home?

The professionals usually will not bombard you with questions, but they will want to make sure that you get what you need and that you feel supported.

It can be hard to make clear and concise decisions when coming out of anesthesia and experiencing a little bit of discomfort. The team members ask questions to get a clear idea of what they can best do to help you move forward and get started on your road to recovery.

YOU
HAVE NOW
COMPLETED
STEP 4

You have now completed step four – the operation itself. What an accomplishment! Congratulations again! You did it! It's over!

All your dreams, all your planning, all your efforts have finally come to fruition - but it's not quite over yet. There are still several steps to consolidate and preserve your efforts in the process of moving forward. First, and perhaps one of the more difficult steps, is that you will have to recover from the trauma of the surgery.

Let's move on to the next step together, Step Five: The Nurturing Process ▦

YOUR **NOTES**

_____

_____

_____

_____

_____

_____

_____

_____

_____

_____

_____

YOUR NOTES

CHAPTER FIVE
STEP FIVE
THE NURTURING PROCESS

THE NURTURING PROCESS

ow hat you have undergone the surgical process, it is time to heal and that brings us to the next step "The Nurturing Process." You have just undergone a surgical procedure, and to recover from it will take a concerted effort on the part of both you and your medical professionals. In our experience, this phase must be conquered with the utmost of care and know-how, with your best interests and comfort taking absolute top priority.

This next section will take you from the operating room to your very own bedroom. This is part of the process where you create what you have visualized. The wisdom shared in this chapter about your recovery process evolved from tried and proven tips from our past patients on the best ways to alleviate your physical discomfort as well as ease any anxieties that might come up during this time of rest.

THE NURTURING PROCESS IS COMPRISED OF **MUCH MORE THAN WHAT WE DO FOR YOU** AFTER YOUR SURGERY. IT IS ABOUT **WHAT YOU DO FOR YOURSELF.**

Staying positive through the entire process is the best preparation for surgery and the best tool for quickly healing afterwards. It is important that you be gentle with yourself. Keep your mind and body healthy and strong. The tools you acquire in this process can help you through what could be a difficult time and serve as valuable skills you can apply to all aspects of your live. The difference between can and cannot is only three letters. Three letters that determine your life's direction.

The nurturing process is comprised of much more than what we do for you after your surgery. It is about what you do for yourself. Your doctor can advise you on what is best, but ultimately you are the one that is going to have to set boundaries and ask for what you need. This is the time when you have to speak up if something isn't working and ask for help if you need it. The nurturing process is really about you offering yourself nurturing.

In your preparation work that you did ahead of the surgery, you already made plans for this process. You took the time and have wisely done a lot of thinking, planning, and preparation for this moment. You have made intricate plans, ranging from your transportation arrangements after the surgery to the smallest aftercare details. It is now time to put these plans into motion. It is time to trust yourself and know that you can do this. It is also time to trust those people that you have asked to help you.

INDIVIDUALIZED
CARE

I f you have been administered anesthesia for your procedure, then you need to have someone drive you home after the surgery. The properties of anesthesia, even in the mildest of forms, can cause several different kinds of immediate side effects. Anesthesia impacts everyone uniquely and some common consequences include drowsiness and confusion. This is why it is important that you don't drive yourself home and that you have a reliable adult who is prepared to watch over you.

Even days after your procedure, it will be important for you to use the utmost care when you start to drive again. Only you can determine when you feel ready to start driving again, but it shouldn't be until after your medical caregivers release you. It will be important that you use clarity and good judgment before getting behind the wheel.

Once you are home, the comforts of familiarity await you. Studies have shown that patients recover best when they return to the coziness of their own home. Perhaps because patients sleep better and are most happy in their own homes, patients recover more quickly, experience less pain and heal faster with fewer infections when they recuperate at home. Upon arriving home, you may have pain or discomfort. Keep in mind that post-operative or incisional pain is normal and it is real. Many surgeons use a local anesthetic to dampen the soreness for a few hours after the surgery is over, but there are other things that you can do once you get home to help decrease pain and swelling.

Use an ice pack on incision sites. This will help keep swelling down and this will also minimize pain as well. You can either use crushed ice in plastic bags, pre-made ice packs, wash cloths that have been soaking in ice water, or even a bag of frozen peas for convenience sake. Frozen peas conform nicely to the face, creating a custom form-fitting ice pack.

Get lots of rest. Your body needs to start the healing process. The more you are able to rest, the more your body can focus on healing and help you feel better.

Keep your head elevated. This is going to help keep the swelling down and will speed up the recovery process. This can be difficult for the first few days and a bit uncomfortable. Many patients choose to sleep on a recliner rather than their bed for the first few days after surgery. If sleeping is a problem you can take medication to help you sleep. Please check with your medical team first before taking an over-the-counter sleeping aid. Some doctors prefer not to prescribe a sleeping aid or sedative for 24 hours following the administration of anesthesia.

Sleep alone. This might not sound like what you want, but it is safer to sleep alone for the first few days after your procedure. You never know when a sleeping partner could bump you in the night, causing you not only pain, but potential injury. It is better that you have your own space to start off the healing process.

Use the medication you have been given. You will have access to pain relief medication. You don't have to be in pain. If your pain levels are too high, use the medication that you have been given. Most patients experience discomfort for the first two to three days after their procedure. Rather than "pain," many describe the sensation after facial surgery as one of pressure, snugness and tightness. Few patients experience the type of stabbing, biting pain that is typical of surgery performed upon other body areas such as the breast, body or tummy.

Be prepared for the discomfort. Having psychological awareness that discomfort is likely can often help it to be more bearable. Don't worry about the pain because it can be treated; just knowing that it is possible can make it easier to deal with.

Be prepared for pressure and tightness. Many patients do not complain of pain after facial surgery. Most patients note pressure, snugness and tightness. Although not considered "pain" in the common sense, your pain medication will help alleviate this discomfort.

Keep your wounds clean and freshly dressed. Certain procedures will require the wounds to be undressed for a specific amount of time. This is to allow for your medical team to observe the incision sites and to allow for drainage. At some point you will have dressings on your incisions. This could be anything from a simple band-aid gauze fixture to your entire head being swathed in bandages. No matter what your dressings, it is important that they are kept clean, dry, and fresh. Every surgeon has his or her own preferred method of performing wound care and applying dressings. You will be given clear instructions on when and how your dressings should be changed. It is imperative to your healing that these instructions are followed.

Keep in mind that bathing may or may not be allowed after your procedure. This will mainly depend on what type of surgery you received. Most often you will be allowed to bathe a couple of days after your procedure, but again, this will depend on the type of surgery. This is another example of the importance of following the directions that you have been given. Not following these instructions can lead to complications and potential damage to your surgical sites.

It is also essential to realize that you may not feel like yourself again, physically, mentally, and emotionally, for several weeks. Expect to have – and enjoy – a nap (or a couple of them) for the next month or so. We heal while we sleep. Expect your emotions to be heightened. Expect some amount of forgetfulness. This is also normal and you will shift back to your old self as you continue to heal. Your body has been through quite an ordeal and it takes time for you to recover from that process and start to feel like yourself again.

Surgeons often blame this fatigue on the anesthesia, but the reality is that it is more likely a combination of the drugs and your body repairing itself. As a result, now is the time to pamper yourself. Indeed, this is your time to focus solely on you. Women are accustomed to being the provider and the nurturer, but now the focus is on pampering and nurturing yourself. After all, you deserve it.

DIETARY
CONSIDERATIONS

art of your pre-planning process was to create a meal schedule for yourself. Ideally when you get home you will not have to cook for yourself, but rather you will have help and support in getting meals made for you.

When you first get home you might not feel hungry. This is not uncommon, especially when the effects of anesthesia are still lingering in your system. Potentially the anesthesia could be making you feel nauseous. Nevertheless, it is important that you eat. You will need some nourishment for strength and sustenance to give your body the energy it requires to start healing.

It is a good idea to start off with something soft and easy to eat. Often patients have soup or yogurt for their first meal after arriving home. At this stage it is also beneficial to drink plenty of liquids (no alcohol, please!). If you have had work done around your mouth, jaw, or cheeks you might have to restrict the amount of chewing that you do. This is another reason to start your food intake with something soft and easy to eat. Because protein is so important for the body's healing process, you might consider an egg when you think you can manage it.

As you recover from your facial plastic surgery, you will definitely want to avoid chewing hard foods. The facial movement required to chew hard foods could aggravate your fresh wounds. Make smart choices and you will notice that you begin to feel stronger and healthier soon.

EMOTIONAL HEALING

t must be said again, when you get home, you will need to rest. It will be important that you find peace and quiet in order for your recovery to get off to a good start. A saying in surgical recovery is, "The strain in pain lies mainly in the brain." This means that you need to be gentle with yourself. This will allow the convalescence period to begin.

Undue emotional stresses will be counterproductive to your main goal, which is a quick and total recovery as soon as possible. After all, you have come this far, so why not take it easy – just for a while longer, anyway. Any feelings of guilt for taking this time for yourself should be cast aside immediately. The more you take care of yourself during this time, the faster you will be able to return to your daily routine and to the ones who love you so dearly. The time you invest in your recovery process will pay off in the long run with a quicker and unrestricted return to your every day activities.

During this time, the focus is on you. Mentally establish the fact that you have just gone through not only a major life change, but also all the accompanying mental anxiety that comes with such an event. This is true even for the many weeks and months prior to the actual procedure. All of the preparation that you have done, from the very first moment of conception to the present, has had its moments of butterflies, concerns, forebodings, misgivings, uncertainties, restlessness, excitement – you name it. So, please, give yourself some space. This is your time to air out, to reflect and to recuperate.

Everyone does this differently; there really isn't one method that works for all individuals. You will need to find both your own way and routine that best fit you and your needs. The main idea is to find some sort of regular system that will allow you to take it easy, feel comfortable, rest your body and mind, and heal.

There is quite a bit of healing to be done, not only physically, but also mentally. Physically you will initially have the usual swelling and bruising that typically results from a major facial plastic surgical procedure. When you first look at yourself in the mirror you may be frightened by what you see. You must remember that bruising, swelling, and other surgical effects will start to fade and disappear quite rapidly. Most often patients see these issues fading within the first two weeks of recovery.

Many find that a little "beauty makeover" can help during this time. Getting simple camouflage makeup can easily hide any noticeable bruises or other obvious results from the surgical procedure. However, these methods should not even be considered until at least eight to ten days after the surgery. We recommend that only professionals properly trained in after-surgery aesthetic care of the cosmetic surgery patient apply these cover-up methods. In many practices, such as our own, this care is supervised by full time medical aestheticians. Our in-house doctor supervised aesthetic staff ensures not only the best possible results but also recommends only safe products that will not irritate your skin.

DURING THIS TIME, **THE FOCUS IS YOU.** MENTALLY ESTABLISH THE FACT THAT YOU HAVE JUST GONE THROUGH NOT ONLY **A MAJOR LIFE CHANGE**, BUT ALL THE ACCOMPANYING **MENTAL ANXIETY** THAT COMES WITH SUCH AN EVENT.

GETTING BACK
TO LIFE

another important part of your recovery process will be the mental preparation for your getting back to your normal routine. This should be a slow and gradual process, but it still needs to be part of your process. You will need to return to your active life with your family, friends, and co-workers. You will need to start thinking about how you are going to start mixing with people with your new appearance. You will need to start thinking about how you are going to react to comments. The best suggestion that we can offer is for you to just be yourself and trust that everything will come together as it should. Keep in mind that you are far more focused on the post-surgical changes than the people that you will encounter. You may think every lump and bump is glaringly obvious, but most folks probably won't notice anything at all.

During your healing time, it is important to keep in mind that your emotions will be running very high. One look in the mirror and all kinds of mental and emotional reactions could be triggered. These reactions cannot be ignored and must be brought to the forefront in order to deal with them directly and play a part in your speedy recovery. Discuss your feelings and discomfort with your friends and family as well as your doctor and his team.

Many patients report that they feel like they are on an emotional roller coaster with their minds racing, full of doubts and fears. One of the stronger emotional thoughts that many patients experience is whether or not they did the right thing. It is not uncommon for people to wonder whether or not their immediate family is going to accept their new look. Many find themselves worrying if their family and friends will like their new look or if they will be rejected. These can be scary and difficult questions to face. Rest assured that many of our patients have felt just like you as they've traveled their recovery path yet they emerged feeling and looking better than ever with very few regrets.

Oftentimes immediate family members will have already expressed strong opposition for facial plastic surgery. The reasons behind their opposition often boil down to loving you the way you are and being scared of you changing. If you exercise patience and understanding, they will eventually come to the realization that your intentions are sincere and genuine. They will start to see that you want to grow into yourself as opposed to trying to be someone else.

Concerns about how your friends will react can also create anxieties. Questions like:

What will they think about the bandages on your face?

How will they react to the swelling and bruising?

What will they say and will they gossip?

Will they think you have changed for the better or for the worse?

What will they think of you, as you have spent so much time, money, and effort on yourself as opposed to others?

Will they still be your friends after all is said and done?

If these people were truly your friends before your surgery, they will certainly be your friends afterwards. If a friend no longer wants to be in a relationship with you because you have made changes to your outward appearance, then he or she was never your real friend to begin with.

Emotions can play tricks on anybody, and right after something as momentous and indelible as your surgery, you are particularly vulnerable. Emotional energy can take a toll on your recovery when facing the prospect of returning to work and dealing with co-workers. In the beginning many patients express great hesitation and reluctance towards returning to the workplace. This is most often connected to worries about what their co-workers and superiors will think of their new look.

As normal as these feelings may be, many are unfounded. Remember, facial plastic surgery often produces subtle results. These results are going to simply enhance the way you look as opposed to change the way you look. Thus, you will simply be producing a better version of yourself instead of a complete metamorphosis of yourself. Rest assured that you look great and your colleagues will be respectful, and perhaps even envious, of your decision to undergo appearance enhancement surgery.

Many of these worries and anxieties are, no doubt, exaggerated due to the rather delicate state that you are in right now. Inevitably the majority of these worries and fears will subside as soon as you start seeing the positive results of your endeavors. As you recognize the beauty of your results, your doubts and fears will diminish. With time, they will vanish into the rear view mirror of the past. Research shows that as time passes, most patients report that they only vaguely remember the anxieties that rattled about in their minds during those early days of recovery.

EMOTIONAL ENERGY CAN TAKE A TOLL ON YOUR RECOVERY WHEN FACING THE PROSPECT OF RETURNING TO WORK AND DEALING WITH CO-WORKERS. IN THE BEGINNING MANY PATIENTS EXPRESS GREAT HESITATION AND RELUCTANCE TOWARDS RETURNING TO THE WORKPLACE.

EXPECTATIONS
AND RISKS

t is important to talk about, and be aware of, some of the consequences of cosmetic surgery. It is appropriate to bring up this information here as we are discussing the healing process. If you know what to expect, you will be better prepared to accept the outcomes of your facial plastic surgery. But, it is important to mention that many of these risks can be avoided by following your instructions for post-operative care. When you take care of yourself after your surgical procedure you are much less likely to have any issues, complications, or problems. As we said in the very first chapter, The Knowledge Builder, knowledge is power and having information about risks can keep you healthy.

The following is a list of the seven most common facial plastic surgery procedures and the risks that are associated with them. This information is intended for general education purposes only and should not be relied upon as a substitute for professional and/or medical advice.

RHINOPLASTY

lso known as a nose job, this cosmetic procedure is used to improve the size, proportion, and overall appearance of your nose. Rhinoplasty will often be combined with septoplasty and perhaps sinus surgery to improve nasal and sinus function and your ability to breathe. Septoplasty is the surgical procedure that straightens the nasal septum, the partition that divides the right side of the nose from the left side of the nose. Septoplasty may be performed alone to correct a deviated nasal septum to improve breathing and sinus function. Septoplasty is very often performed at the same time as a rhinoplasty. As with all surgery, perhaps the most important factor in achieving a great and complication-free result is choosing an experienced special-ist in rhinoplasty. A board certified facial plastic surgeon is an expert in rhinoplasty, septoplasty and septorhinoplasty. Here are some of the risks that are involved with getting a rhinoplasty procedure:

Infection: This can happen at the incision sites. It is rare and will most often heal with antibiotics.

Poor healing: If you don't take care of the incision sites, poor healing can result. This can lead to noticeable scars and the potential for necessary follow-up surgical procedures.

Spider vein formation affecting the nasal skin: The vessels of the nose can rupture, but it is a rare occurrence. This can lead to discoloration, failure of the procedure and necessary follow-up procedures.

Bleeding: Although a certain amount of bleeding is to be expected, serious bleeding that can lead to long term issues is very rare. Occasionally, the nose may need to be packed with surgical sponges to control bleeding.

Nose asymmetry: Occasionally a rhinoplasty can leave the nose looking asymmetrical. An ideal, symmetric nose is uncommon. It is uncommon that a nose is ideal or perfectly symmetric prior to surgery and so therefore, it is impractical to expect that the post-surgical result will be 'perfect.' Although we aim to achieve perfection and the ideal nose, it is unrealistic to expect that this will be achieved.

Numbness or other changes in sensation: Anytime surgery is performed there is a risk of numbness or changes in sensation. This is due to the surgical procedure itself, and although some numbness is normal, it will generally go away on its own. Sometimes the upper front teeth may also be numb for some time after surgery. Permanent numbness is rare.

Septum perforation: The septum is the partition that separates the right and left nasal passages from one another. Perforation of the nasal septum occurs when a hole is punctured in the center of the nasal passage. This can lead to nasal whistling, bleeding and breathing problems. Subsequent repair of the nasal septal perforation may be necessary if the problem persists.

Scarring: A certain amount of scarring will happen, but most often it is not noticeable. Sometimes, massage will help diminish swelling. Injection of certain medications after surgery may be needed to control and lessen scarring if present.

Blockage of the air passages: When working around the nose there is always some risk of blocking the air passages. This is uncommon and can be corrected with a follow up procedure.

Ongoing pain: Some amount of pain is to be expected, but if pain is persistent, this is something you will want to discuss with your medical team.

Skin irregularities: After a procedure there will be some amount of changes to the skin, but it is often unnoticeable and dissipates with time in most cases.

Discoloration: Some amount of skin discoloration will typically fade a few months after the procedure.

Potential for follow-up surgical procedures: Many of the above complications can require follow-up procedures. Additional rhinoplasty procedures are considered more complicated. In general, experience shows that about ten percent of rhinoplasty patients will seek a second, revisional or refinement procedure.

As a reminder, closely following your surgeon's post-procedure instructions as they will help you from encountering any of these unfavorable results. It is important not to press upon or manipulate your nose as you recover from surgery. The nasal bones and cartilage can be moved and reshaped for six weeks or more after surgery. This means that if you were to push hard, firmly massage, wear heavy glasses or goggles or fall upon your nose that you could move the nose and change its shape or cause it to become crooked.

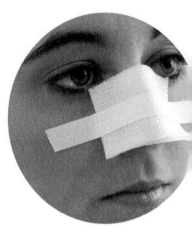

EYELID SURGERY

yelid surgery is technically called a blepharoplasty. This procedure rejuvenates the upper and lower lids of both eyes to create a more youthful and rejuvenated look. Eyelid blepharoplasty is a meticulous surgical procedure. To reduce your risk and to help ensure that you achieve your desired result, be certain to choose an experienced surgeon who performs blepharoplasty often and is a specialist in eyelid and facial plastic surgery. Below you will find some of the risks that you need to be aware of when considering blepharoplasty.

Scarring: The incision for upper eyelid surgery is hidden within the upper eyelid crease where the eyelid folds upon itself. Oftentimes, the lower eyelid incision can be placed invisibly within the internal surface of the lower eyelid rather than in the skin itself. With time, eyelid blepharoplasty incisions generally heal very well. Unfavorable scarring is uncommon. Less than optimal incisions can often be treated with a laser to improve their appearance. As long as your surgeon properly places the incision, eyelid scars usually fade away rather nicely.

Blurred or impaired vision that may or may not be permanent: While working around the eyes there are a number of problems that can cause impaired vision. This is not uncommon for a short while after your surgery and most often clears up after a few days recovery. Permanent alteration of vision, although a risk, is fortunately quite rare.

Dry eyes: Eye dryness is normal for some time after eyelid surgery and will commonly clear up after a few days to weeks. Eye drops and lubricating eye ointment are often suggested around the time of surgery to relieve discomfort from the dryness.

Difficulty closing the eyes: Rarely the eyes are drawn too tightly and closing the eyes is difficult. Occasionally this could require follow up procedures. Usually this will relax with time and be passing in nature.

Lid lag or a pulling down of the lower eyelid: Rarely the eyes can be adjusted so the lid doesn't function properly or there is a hanging of the lower eyelid. This will occasionally require follow up procedures. Many surgeons prefer placing the incision inside the lower eyelid, known as transconjunctival blepharoplasty, because it better maintains the position and shape of the lower eyelid.

Bruising and Bleeding: Some amount of bruising is to be expected. Significant bleeding can be dangerous and could cause issues with vision. It is important to avoid blood thinners, lifting and straining after surgery to minimize the likelihood of unexpected bleeding after surgery.

Poor healing: When post-procedural care is not followed, the wound may not heal properly.

Infection: Issues with infection are rare and are most often treated with antibiotics.

Fluid accumulation: Puffiness and fluid can accumulate after surgery. This can be minimized with elevation, ice and avoidance of salty and higher sodium food and drink after surgery.

Numbing or skin changes: There will be some amount of numbness and skin changes after a procedure, but these tend to fade with time.

Complications from anesthesia: There are always potential issues from receiving anesthesia. These are rare and unlikely when the patient is in good health.

Ongoing pain: Some amount of discomfort is to be expected, but if the pain is more than you expect, doesn't respond to pain medication, or goes on for too long, make sure that you report this to your medical team. Significant pain after eyelid surgery is uncommon and should alert you and your medical team to look for a problem.

Swelling and discoloration: There will be a certain amount of swelling and discoloration. This should fade within a couple of weeks after the procedure.

It is vitally important that you follow the recommendations of your medical team after your procedure. This will help minimize the possibility of complications and allow your healing process to be smooth and easy.

FACELIFT

facelift is medically referred to as a rhytidectomy and it is one of the more common facial cosmetic procedures performed. Although it takes longer to recover from this procedure than some of the other options, the changes are dramatic and long lasting. As with any medical procedure there are a certain amount of risks and complications that can occur. Facelift is a specialized procedure that requires concentration and artistic skill on the part of the surgeon. To achieve a natural and youthful appearance, select an experienced surgeon who specializes in facelift surgery as a major part of his or her practice. Below you will find some of the potential issues that you might run into when getting a facelift procedure.

Scarring: Whenever an incision is created, a scar results. The key is for the scar to be made unnoticeable. Facelift incisions are commonly placed beginning within the temple hair or sideburn, then within the crease that lies in front of the ear and then behind the ear and again into the hairline. With time, facelift incisions generally heal very well. Unfavorable scarring is uncommon. Less than optimal incisions can often be treated with a laser to improve their appearance.

Bleeding: A certain amount of bleeding and bruising is to be expected after a facelift procedure, but this should be minimal. Serious bleeding is rare and should be reported to your medical team immediately. If you feel sudden or progressive swelling, fullness or tightness, this should also be reported as soon as possible to your surgeon.

Infection: The facial region has such a strong blood supply that infection in and around the face, head and neck is unlikely. If infection does occur, it is typically easy to treat. Antibiotics prescribed around the time of your surgery may decrease the likelihood of infection after your procedure.

Poor wound healing: If you follow all of the post-procedural instruction poor wound healing should not be an issue. This is an uncommon problem and most often occurs in smokers and when patients don't follow instructions carefully.

Complications from anesthesia: There are always potential issues from receiving anesthesia. These are rare and unlikely when the patient is in good health.

Hair loss at incision sites: There is often some amount of hair loss that will happen from this procedure, but most often the hair grows back with few issues.

Facial asymmetry: A rare issue that can develop after a facelift. Most often, facial asymmetry will sort itself out as swelling subsides; but on the rare occasion follow-up procedures might be necessary.

Nerve injury: Any time the skin is cut there is some amount of nerve damage. Most often this repairs itself and as long as no major nerves were damaged the injury is temporary. Permanent nerve damage rarely occurs.

Skin loss or skin necrosis: When incisions are made into the skin there is always the possibility of skin necrosis. This is when the blood flow is restricted and the skin starts to die and fall off. This is very rare and tends to happen more often in patients that smoke.

Numbness or change in sensation: Following a surgical procedure there will be a certain amount of numbness or change in sensation. This is usually temporary and normal sensation returns as swelling decreases, typically within a few days to a couple of weeks.

Fluid accumulation: On the rare occasion fluid can accumulate under the skin. This often resolves itself after a couple of days and can be avoided when proper measures have been taken to ensure drainage of the incision sites. At times, such a fluid accumulation may need to be drained and a snug pressure bandage applied to aid in healing and to prevent re-accumulation of the fluid.

Discoloration: There will be a certain amount of skin discoloration, but this is most often temporary and will resolve itself over the first few days to weeks of healing. There are a number of things to do to prevent bruising such as avoiding blood thinners and certain medications and vitamins around the time of surgery. Your surgical team should advise you accordingly in this regard. There are also some special techniques such as lymphatic massage and drainage that can help this resolve. Certain vitamins, homeopathic remedies and topical creams can help bruising resolve more quickly, but such products should be started only with the expressed approval and supervision of your surgical team.

Deep venous thrombosis: DVT is a serious medical complication that can occur with prolonged surgical procedures, during periods of immobility and in individuals with blood clotting disorders and a personal or family history of such disorders. It is important to communicate this history to your medical and anesthesia team. Certain precautions can be taken during your surgery to reduce this risk. Getting up out of bed and walking as soon as you are comfortable and safe after surgery may reduce this risk. Fortunately, DVT is much less common with facial, head and neck surgery than it is with surgery on other body sites.

Potential for follow up procedures being needed: As with any surgical procedure the potential for a follow up or touch up to improve an unexpected problem may prove necessary. Although uncommon, generally in less than ten percent of cases, an enhancement procedure is often minor and, at times, can be accomplished rather simply.

It is important to follow the post-operative instructions that have been provided to you. Be gentle with yourself after the procedure. Get lots of rest in order to fully recover with as few complications or potential risks as possible.

∨ BEFORE; Actual Patient Browlift

∨ AFTER; Actual Patient Browlift

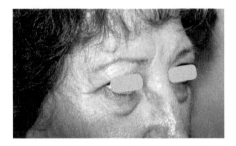
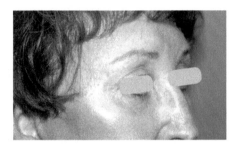

BROWLIFT

a browlift or a forehead lift is done to decrease the amount of lines and wrinkles on the forehead. The lift will reposition the brow and get rid of any sagging. Brow lift and forehead lift also act to smooth horizontal forehead lines and the 'vertical 11's' between the brows. As with any cosmetic procedure there are some complications and risks that can happen. Facial plastic surgeons are specialists who focus on this sort of surgery and because of their experience achieve excellence in brow and forehead plastic surgery. Below you will find some of the risks that you should be aware of before getting a brow lift procedure.

Scarring: Some amount of scarring is going to be the reality of any surgical procedure, but it should be unnoticeable.

Bleeding: Although a certain amount of bleeding is to be expected, serious bleeding that can lead to permanent problems is very rare.

Infection: Issues with infection are rare and are most often treated with a simple round of antibiotics.

Poor wound healing: If you follow all of the post-procedural instructions, poor wound healing should not be an issue. This is a rare problem and most often occurs when patients don't follow instructions.

Complications from anesthesia: There are always potential issues from receiving anesthesia. These are rare and unlikely when the patient is in good health.

Blood clotting: This is a potentially serious issue, but it is also rare. Blood clotting is recorded in less than one percent of procedures.

Hair loss at incision sites: There is often some amount of hair loss that will happen from this procedure, but most often the hair grows back with few issues.

Facial nerve damage: Any time the skin is cut there is some amount of nerve damage. Most often this repairs itself and as long as no major nerves were damaged the injury is temporary. Permanent nerve damage rarely occurs.

Facial asymmetry: A rare issue that can develop after a facelift. Most often, facial asymmetry will sort itself out as swelling subsides; but on the rare occasion follow-up procedures might be necessary.

Skin loss or skin necrosis: When incisions are made into the skin there is always the possibility of skin necrosis. This is when the blood flow is restricted and the skin starts to die and fall off. This is very rare and tends to happen more often in patients that smoke.

Change in skin sensation, including numbness or itching: After a cosmetic procedure it is not uncommon for your skin sensations to be different. Most often this fades after a few days healing. If you have issues with itching, numbness, or other sensation changes after a few weeks check in with your medical team.

Eye irritation or dryness: Eye dryness is normal and will clear up after a few days. Eye drops can be used to deal with any discomfort from the dryness.

Accumulation of fluid: On the rare occasion fluid can accumulate under the skin. This often resolves itself after a couple of days and can be avoided when proper measures have been taken to insure drainage of the incision sites.

Ongoing pain: Some amount of pain is to be expected, but if pain is overwhelming or isn't helped with medication, this is something you will want to discuss with your medical team.

Irregularities of skin contour: It is not uncommon for the skin to look and feel different after a plastic surgery procedure. More often than not, these changes are temporary and will subside as healing takes place.

Discoloration: There will be a certain amount of skin discoloration, but this is most often temporary and will resolve itself over the first few days of healing.

Potential need for corrective surgery to be performed: Many of the above complications can require follow up procedures being needed. Additional procedures are considered more risky and have a higher potential for risks.

By following your post-operative care instructions you are less likely to have any of these complications become a serious issue.

LASER SKIN RESURFACING AND DERMABRASION

ermabrasion and laser skin resurfacing stimulate the creation of a new layer of skin that is relatively free of lines, wrinkles and imperfections and is more youthful in appearance. This procedure has very few complications that can happen, but it is good to know what the potential issues could be. The use of a laser requires experience and expertise on the part of the practitioner. It is unfortunate that any doctor can purchase a laser including doctors that have no real experience in facial plastic surgery or cosmetic skin surgery. Below you will find some of the changes that can happen after skin resurfacing and dermabrasion treatments.

Milia and whiteheads: This is a normal reaction to the resurfacing process. Not everyone goes through this phase, but it will often clear up after a few days of healing.

Changes to skin pigmentation: Pinkness of the skin is part of the normal healing process after this procedure. Pinkness tends to be more prominent in fair skin individuals than in darker or more oily skin types. In either case, your normal coloring will return. Sun exposure will prolong the pinkness and can create a very troubling mottling and stubborn dark discoloration of the skin. Careful sun avoidance, use of a reliable sunblock and correct skin care will ensure proper healing.

Enlargement of skin pores: The treatment will often leave your skin open and sensitive. One of the side effects of this procedure is temporarily enlarged skin pores. They will start to close up on their own, but if it bothers you, additional skin care treatments can be done.

Infection: This is a rare issue from this treatment, but still potentially possible. Following the post-treatment instructions can lower the risk of infection. Most infections can be treated with simple antibiotics. Skin resurfacing can also reactivate cold sores. In certain patients and in certain types of resurfacing, antiviral medications may be prescribed. It is very important that you follow these instructions carefully.

Scarring: Highly rare from this procedure, but in very few cases there is some scarring that can happen. This most often occurs when the provider is not well trained or inexperienced or the patient has failed to care for the treated regions properly and according to doctor's instructions.

Following the guidelines on how to care for your skin after the resurfacing procedure will help you avoid any of these issues or complications. This is a remarkably common procedure that should have very few post-procedure issues.

CHEMICAL PEEL

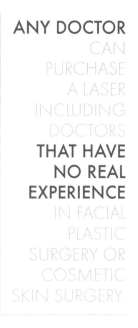

there are several different strengths of chemical peels that can be used to remove wrinkles, fine lines, scars, and discoloration from the top layers of the skin of the face, neck, chest, hands and arms. This system is one of the easiest ways to improve the appearance of the skin. Chemical peel is very similar to mechanical methods of resurfacing such as laser and dermabrasion. The results and healing course are very similar among the procedures. The different options for the depth of a chemical peel are termed very light, light, medium, and deep peels. Some lighter methods of peeling are performed by aestheticians and nurses while the deeper techniques are typically limited to physicians who specialize in facial plastic surgery. Complications can result from any chemical peel treatment though the risks increase with stronger chemical peel options:

ANY DOCTOR CAN PURCHASE A LASER INCLUDING DOCTORS THAT HAVE NO REAL EXPERIENCE IN FACIAL PLASTIC SURGERY OR COSMETIC SKIN SURGERY.

Temporary or permanent color discoloration: There will be a certain amount of skin discoloration, especially with the deep peel options. This is temporary and, as with the lighter peels, will fade after a few days. With the deep peels, skin discoloration can last for several months.

Infection: The stronger the peel the higher the risk of infection, but infection overall is very rare. The best way to avoid infection is to follow directions and take care of your skin after the procedure. If infection becomes an issue it can easily be treated with antibiotics.

Scarring: There is always a risk of scarring with a chemical peel and the stronger the peel the higher the risk. This is a rare issue and the risk of scarring is clearly greater when the practitioner is unskilled.

Activation of cold sores: The chemical peel process can activate the herpes virus. This is, of course, only an issue if you have the herpes virus prior to undergoing the chemical peel procedure.

∨ BEFORE; Actual Patient Chemical Peel   ∨ AFTER; Actual Patient Chemical Peel

Sensitivity to sun: After a chemical peel you will need to be wary of being in the sun. The stronger the peel the longer you will need to be watching your sun exposure levels. This will fade over time, but staying out of the sun will also help the effects of your procedure last longer.

CHEMICAL PEELS CAN BE USED TO **REMOVE** WRINKLES, FINE LINES, SCARS, AND DISCOLORATION FROM THE TOP LAYERS OF THE **SKIN** OF THE **FACE NECK CHEST HANDS** AND **ARMS**

Redness: There will be redness of the skin after a chemical peel and this is true for all the strength levels. The stronger the peel, the longer the redness will last, but ultimately it is temporary.

Skin crusting: A certain amount of skin crusting or scabbing may happen after a chemical peel, but the goal is to avoid this as much as possible. When you follow the post- procedure instructions and keep your face clean and well moisturized, you should be able to minimize this issue as much as possible.

Stinging: Your skin will be sensitive after a chemical peel and this is often described as a stinging sensation. This will subside as your skin begins to heal and regenerate.

Skin peeling: Some skin peeling is to be expected, as this is a natural part of the sloughing off process. Skin peeling should be temporary; as your new skin starts to come to rest the peeling should stop.

Cysts or white spots: After the peel, especially a deep chemical peel, your skin might develop cysts or white spots. This is much like the milia that we see after dermabrasion or laser skin resurfacing.

The best way to avoid these issues from a chemical peel is to be honest about any scarring issues that you have had in the past. If you have sensitivity to scarring this could lead to a higher likelihood of problems from a chemical peel procedure.

You should receive clear instructions on what you should do after your chemical peel procedure to keep your skin healthy and avoid complications. Following these guidelines is going to help you avoid these risks.

THE INJECTABLES:
RELAXERS AND FILLERS

here are a great many fillers and injectables that have flooded the cosmetic surgery market in the last decade. This trend toward minimally invasive lunchtime treatments is likely to continue well into the future. Common treatments include the muscle relaxers (Botox, Xeomin and Dysport) and the fillers (Restylane, Perlane, Juvederm, Radiesse, Belotero, Sculptra, Artefill and Prevelle). These are popular and successful methods for treating facial lines and wrinkles. Even though the risks and complications are generally minor and pass with time, if improperly performed you could end up with a displeasing result that you are stuck with for many months. Any licensed doctor can treat you with these fillers. There are very few restrictions. Although many types of doctors perform these injections and many patients are motivated by price, it truly is a skill and an art to perform these injections skillfully. A facial plastic surgeon's intimate knowledge of facial anatomy helps achieve a great result. It is important to know the risks in order for you to be properly informed.

Unskilled injector: Perhaps the greatest risk with these treatments is that you will not be pleased with your result. Among the most common complaints after treatment are that the correction does not last, is partial or incomplete, that the filler is uneven, or that the injection was painful or associated with undue bruising. Some of these complications occur because the injector is unskilled or improperly trained. Motivated by price, patients often seek the lowest cost provider assuming that all fillers are the same and so the lowest priced place is the way to go. This is often shortsighted and results in months of unhappiness. Be certain that you seek a skilled facial plastic surgeon.

Bruising of the injection site: Whenever an injection is performed, whether it is the flu shot, drawing a blood sample, or an injectable cosmetic skin treatment, there is a risk of bruising at the treatment site. This is a common occurrence and will often clear up within a few days of treatment. Makeup can often be applied immediately following your treatment. Ice, elevation and certain creams and vitamins may help bruising resolve.

Swelling at the injection site: This is a common side effect from the injections and will often clear up within a few hours. If you experience a lot of swelling or it lasts for more than a week, you should consult your medical team.

Pain at the injection site: As with any injection, there is some discomfort. Fortunately, the needles used with cosmetic injectables are among the finest and smallest available in all of medicine. If you experience ongoing pain, you should check in with your medical team.

Redness: Some amount of redness is normal after an injectable treatment. This will fade anywhere from a few hours to a few days after the injections.

Headache: This is another common side effect after a filler treatment. This will most likely fade within a few hours of the treatment. It may be related to the stress and anticipation of your treatment rather than to the product itself. If your headache persists for longer than a few days, check with your medical team.

Flu symptoms: Some patients remark upon very minor flu-like symptoms after some of the relaxers (Botox, Dysport and Xeomin). This issue most often clears up on its own within a few days of the procedure and typically does not require any treatment.

Facial asymmetry: A rare issue that can develop after a facelift. Most often, facial asymmetry will sort itself out as swelling subsides; but on the rare occasion follow-up procedures might be necessary.

t is important after a relaxer or filler treatment to not rub or massage the treated areas unless specifically instructed to do so by your practitioner. This can lead to the toxin spreading into other areas of your face, which, in turn, can lead to drooping or weakness. In the case of filler, it can lead to unwanted spreading of the filler product, creating lumpiness and unevenness.

After your injectable treatment you can return to your regular life right away. If you follow the directions that we give to you after the procedure, you are less likely to have problems or complications. Relaxers and fillers are safe and any complications or risks that do occur tend to be temporary. As the relaxer and filler fade out of the system, these complications fade as well.

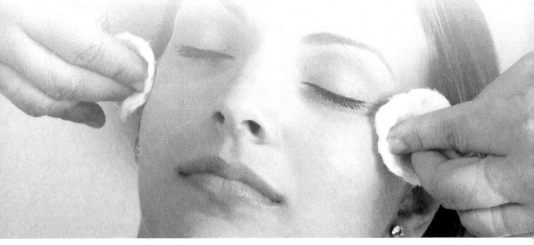

IMPORTANT WORDS
ABOUT SMOKING

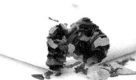

he use of tobacco adversely affects all aspects of an individual's health and well-being and smoking is problematic in facial plastic surgery as well. Patients should be aware that smoking and tobacco of all sorts impair wound healing while causing significant adverse outcomes. It also increases the complication rate in elective facial plastic surgery and in facial cosmetic surgery. It is recommended the patient stop smoking for a minimum of two weeks, and preferably four weeks, prior to the surgical procedure and to remain tobacco-free for a minimum of two weeks, and preferably four weeks, after the surgical procedure. Patients who are not willing to stop smoking around the time of their surgery have higher rates of morbidity and complications.

In smokers, there is an increased risk of postoperative pulmonary problems, including, but not limited to, skin loss or necrosis, bruising, bleeding, flap impairment, delayed wound healing, scarring, and loss of hair that could be permanent and significantly compromise the outcome of the procedure. There are benefits of seeking a professional counselor, if needed, to stop smoking. Nicotine substitutes, such as inhalers, patches, and gums, are unacceptable around the time of your surgery as these drugs and devices also impair wound healing.

In my practice, I discuss with each patient how the use of tobacco adversely affects all aspects of their health and well-being and is problematic in facial plastic surgery. I inform each patient that it impairs wound healing, causing significant adverse outcomes, and increases the complication rate in elective facial plastic surgery and in facial cosmetic surgery. I ask my patients to sign an informed consent form acknowledging that they understand the risks of smoking relative to facial surgery.

IN SUMMARY

t bears repeating that taking care of yourself after your procedure and following all of the care guidelines is going to help prevent many of these risks from becoming an issue. Selecting a skilled specialist in facial plastic surgery who is an expert in these procedures and performs them often should also help ensure a complication-free outcome. Knowing the risks is important because it gives you clear information to help you make an informed decision. However, worrying about potential risks isn't worth it. Just follow the post-op guidelines, take care of yourself, and relax.

DURING **RECOVERY**

here are many things that you might normally do to relax that may not be allowed after a cosmetic procedure. Your physical activities will need to be reduced as rest and relaxation becomes the priority. Since you won't be able to do some of your typical activities, you might start looking at some other things to keep you occupied and entertained as you heal. The following list is some things that you might consider, during your healing process.

SPIRITUAL PURSUITS

ne way that you might consider this is by reading scriptural texts, spiritual books, or books pertaining to some form of divine inspiration. These types of pursuits can serve as a very effective catalyst for one's prompt recovery.

If your reading has been restricted during your recovery process, you will want to consider getting books on tape to help you get the spiritual insight without putting strain on your eyes.

YOGA

oga is a popular activity for many, and regular practitioners claim very positive results through overall improved general health. Hatha Yoga concentrates on physical positioning and is recognized as a very compelling way to reduce stress and obtain a sense of well-being. This should be reserved for people who are already somewhat versed in the art of yogic postures. Any physical strain that you undergo at this time would be counterproductive, so caution should be adhered to. Focus should be on the less stressful and more relaxing yogic postures and states. If you are looking to take a yoga class during your healing process, explain to the instructor that you've just undergone surgery and get their advice on which positions you should pursue.

MEDITATION AND PRAYER

editation is an excellent practice for calming your mind, quieting your worries, and finding that inner place of calm and ease. People from cultures all over the world use meditation as a means of finding spiritual enlightenment, quieting the mind, and taking some time away from the world by going within and getting to the calm place that we all have inside of us. Meditation can be done with tapes, videos, or on your own. There are also many meditation groups that meet and can help you to develop your own meditation practice.

Another form of meditation is prayer. Many patients consider prayer to be the active form of meditation. During prayer you focus your thoughts and emotions on something outside of yourself. This might be a higher power or it might be your loved ones. Prayer can be done on your own or with the use of prayer beads, mandalas, or other objects to help you focus your prayer and quiet your mind from distracting thoughts. Meditation and prayer can help you to calm your emotions, quiet your mind, and go to a place that is beyond yourself. For many people healing from surgery, this is one of the best ways to start feeling better and stop worries from taking over.

READING

eading is another great way to convalesce. Even light reading can work wonders for the mind and be very relaxing. Many patients have reported that self-help books, primers on hobbies, and even some of the best fiction books not only aid in passing time, but also contribute to helping one grow in many different and intangible ways.

There are a lot of so-called "New Age" bestsellers that seem to be flying off the shelves these days. Such popular writings as The Alchemist, by Paulo Coelho, The Prophet, by Khalil Gibran, The Secret, by Rhonda Bryne and Seven Spiritual Laws of Success, by Deepak Chopra all lend insights towards spiritual growth in our contemporary society.

Newspapers and magazines also offer valued time for thought and reflection. Oprah Winfrey's magazine "O" puts forward insightful and provocative interviews by very successful people whose viewpoints are greatly valued by men and women alike from all walks of life. Find a magazine that keeps your interest and keeps your mind occupied. Electronic readers such as the Kindle, Nook and iPad are great as you recover. With access to the internet, these devices allow infinite reading and video options without ever leaving your home. This is a particularly attractive option since, as you finish a book, newspaper or magazine, another issue can be on your reader in moments without ever leaving the house. Reading not only furnishes an opportunity to remain quiet and restful, but it also presents great challenges for the mind.

WATCH A MOVIE

eading may require too much concentration or focus as you recover and everyone loves a great movie. We live in an amazing era of technology. With high speed internet, laptops and tablets, movies can stream to your favorite device at your every whim. Whether you're in the mood for an oldie or a new release, a comedy or a love story or just reruns of your favorite sitcom or drama, download the show and catch up as you recover. This is a great way to unwind and tune out as your body heals from your recent surgery.

REST, REST, REST

f you tend to be an active and energetic person you may find that this time of quietude is not easy to sustain. For many patients, by their very nature, relaxing is not in their vocabulary. For these people, recovery from facial plastic surgery is generally prolonged. This is often because they get involved with physical activity too soon after surgery. But "rest, rest, rest" has different definitions for every individual. Resting might include reading, watching movies, crossword puzzles, Sudoku, meditation and prayer. There are also so many great internet options such as playing virtual Scrabble with players worldwide. Consider some of these opportunities before your surgery.

If you have a regular workout routine, are an avid hiker, or take part in some other vigorous physical activity, it is imperative that you take a break while you are healing. Pushing yourself to resume physical activities too soon can have detrimental effects on your healing. Taking time out from exercise can mean the difference between a clean and smooth healing as opposed to infection and scarring. The time you invest in rest and relaxation around the time of your surgery will reward you in a quicker recovery.

RESTING MIGHT INCLUDE READING, WATCHING MOVIES, CROSSWORD PUZZLES, SUDOKU, MEDITATION AND PRAYER. CONSIDER SOME OF THESE OPPORTUNITIES BEFORE YOUR SURGERY.

This leads me to talk about some precautions that I feel compelled to explain. Most of these are based on common sense, but it is important to remember these things for a smooth and easy healing process. Remember that some simple physical activities are serious no-nos after your cosmetic procedure. Picking up your child might seem harmless and easy, but if your precious baby bumps your newly formed nose, this can have a major impact on how you heal.

I cannot say it enough; this process is about you. In order to have the look that we have both worked so hard to achieve, you need to give yourself the time and space to heal. What this really means is:

NO LIFTING - Lifting anything, no matter how light the object may be, should be kept to an absolute minimum. Any kind of straining to lift something, including little children, may have an adverse effect on your new surgery. Lift nothing heavier than a phone book until otherwise instructed by your doctor.

NO HOUSEWORK - Even something as simple as running a vacuum, bending to empty the dishwasher, loading clothes into the washer and dryer could very easily compromise your wounds.

NO BENDING - Bending over forces blood and fluid to flow towards your face. This is something that you don't want especially right after your surgery. It will be important for you to avoid leaning over, bending over, and doing anything that causes blood to flow into the top of your body.

NO DRIVING - At least for the first few weeks after your surgery you should not be driving. There is too much that can go wrong behind the wheel of the car. You don't want to compromise your whole surgery just to get some ice cream do you? Most accidents happen within four blocks of someone's home, so better to avoid the possibility until it is safer.

W hat about exercise?' you might be asking. Exercise is good as long as you don't overdo it! You need to be sure that you ease into exercising slowly and gradually - and I really mean gradually. You may be de-conditioned after your surgery and will find that you don't have the same level of stamina after your procedure. Take your time working back up to the daily exercise routine that you had before your plastic surgery. Vigorous workouts can be very counterproductive because they raise your blood pressure. Increased blood pressure can result in excess blood to the face, swelling, and even bleeding.

This is why if you are a jogger, for example, you will need to start getting back into jogging very slowly. Instead of going for a run, you might consider simply walking your route for a number of days (or even weeks) before you start any of the jerky motions that running places on your body. You may even want to play on the safe side and forego any running at all until healing is complete.

All aerobic exercise should be treated like jogging. If you take a spin class, a workout class, or other type of exercise to get your heart rate going, you should really take a long break and let your healing process be your main focus. Exercise will still be there when you are healed and it will be easy for you to get back into shape and back into your normal routine.

Weightlifting needs to be avoided until your healing is complete. Lifting weights puts pressure on your body and causes you to strain. This is something that you do not want to be doing while you are healing. It is good to wait several months before adding weightlifting back into your exercise routine. As with any other exercise, you need to check with your medical team before starting your weightlifting practice back up.

Pilates is one form of exercise that you might be able to move back into sooner, although you still need to be careful. Pilates can cause you to strain your body, which is pressure that you do not want to have. It also works with slow and deliberate movements, which can help you to get exercise without hurting yourself. It is better to be safe than sorry so make sure that you check in with your medical care team before going back to a Pilates routine.

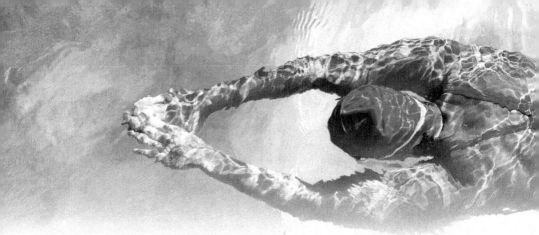

Swimming is a similar issue. Chlorinated pool water or salty ocean water is often safe for incisions. Fresh water is more likely to bear contaminants. Avoid hot tubs. The key problem with resuming swimming is sun exposure. As discussed below, direct sunlight can cause incisions to become thickened scars and skin to become discolored. Be sure to discuss this with your surgical care team.

Whatever the case, post-operative instructions need to be followed in order to help your healing process and allow for a smoother recovery. Common sense will tell you that moderation should be the norm here, gradually working up to your regular routine. In fact, reasonable exercise will get that blood circulating, keep your ticker going, and give you a general overall feeling of contentment, all aspects of which will expedite the healing process.

SUN EXPOSURE
PROTECT YOUR INVESTMENT

his brings us to the discussion of going outdoors. Getting outside after weeks of inside convalescing can be really refreshing and it can go a long way towards helping you to feel like yourself again. But there are several precautions that you need to seriously consider before taking the first step into the fresh air and sunshine. After all, exposure to the sun can be catastrophic for your new surgery, especially if you have had a full facelift or facial resurfacing. Direct exposure to the sun could lead to irreversible blotchiness or changes in your pigment tones. Sun exposure could even negate the positive results of your surgery entirely.

So yes, get outside and breathe fresh air, but do so smartly, remembering that your new face needs to be protected from the harsh and damaging rays of the sun. Here are a few tips that should be followed for keeping your face safe from the potential damage of the sun. Protecting yourself from the sun isn't just something you need to keep in mind for the weeks and months after your surgery, but for the rest of your life.

▶ **HAT -** For at least six months after surgery, you should wear a wide brimmed hat to protect your face from the sun. The brim should be at least three to four inches all around the hat. In other words, it should be 360 degrees all the way around the hat, not just a visor. A baseball cap does not provide good sun protection. It leaves the lower face, neck and ears fully exposed to the sun. The hat should be made of a tightly woven fabric. Straw hats are generally useless as too much sun passes between the openings in the straw weave. Hats today often come marked with a UPF factor. This is like the SPF label that we see on sun block. Look for the UPF rating as you shop for a hat before your surgery. A hat can make it easy for you to go outside, while keeping yourself protected.

▶ **SUNSCREEN -** For six months after your procedure you should put on sunscreen (SPF 30-plus) before you go outside. This should be applied before you leave the house and re-applied every couple of hours. This will help to minimize the number of extremely damaging ultraviolet rays that will be shining down on your sensitive skin. Makeup with sunblock is usually not sufficient. Look for a sunblock that contains zinc oxide, titanium dioxide or Parsol 1789 to ensure good UVA and UVB sunlight protection.

▶ **AVOID THE SUN -** The best way to avoid sun exposure is to simply not go outside. But this is impractical and not much fun. Go outside and enjoy yourself. Wear a good hat, strong sunblock and when you are outside, try to stay in the shade as much as possible.

Once again, the moderation rule could very easily be applied here: Try to expose yourself to the sun as little as possible. When you are outside in the areas of direct sunshine, it will be important for you to take the appropriate precautions.

SMOKING

d o I need to say anything more about smoking? Maybe not, but I am going to anyway. At this point you should already know how detrimental tobacco products can be both before and after surgery. The facts were reiterated earlier in this chapter and were previously explained in Chapter Three – Step Three – The Preparation and Reassurance Program.

Some surgeons have been known to refuse to perform surgery on patients who will not comply with certain rules and limitations on smoking around the time of surgery. You are certainly fully aware of the damages that the use of tobacco can cause on the human body and the complications that smoking will cause during the operative and post-operative stages of facial plastic surgery.

Poor wound healing, increased risk of infection, longer-lasting bruises, skin necrosis, and raised and thickened scars are just a few of the potential issues, as I have already mentioned. I also realize that smokers have their rights and preferences as well, and I certainly do not refuse any smoker who agrees to follow my stringent rules.

YOU ARE CERTAINLY **FULLY AWARE** OF THE **DAMAGES** THAT THE **USE OF TOBACCO** CAN CAUSE ON THE **HUMAN BODY** AND THE **COMPLICATIONS** THAT **SMOKING WILL CAUSE DURING THE OPERATIVE AND POST-OPERATIVE STAGES OF FACIAL PLASTIC SURGERY.**

To reiterate, smokers also must recognize that cosmetic surgery is an investment and that each patient should participate and do his or her part to ensure the best possible outcome.

Furthermore it is our experience at the Clevens Face and Body Specialists that many patients who quit smoking for four to six weeks in the pre-operative period remain long term non-smokers. Since fewer than one in ten smokers are successful in becoming long term non-smokers, it is our hope, as facial plastic surgery professionals, that we can benefit the health of our patients by encouraging smoking cessation in a positive and supportive fashion.

MEDICATION AND SUPPLEMENTS

ust as your medication regimen should be discussed with your surgeon and his team in detail prior to your surgery, post-operative medication and supplements should be discussed with equal importance. Far too many patients try to self-medicate themselves after the surgery and end up causing severe reactions and complications as a result. There are a lot of misconceptions as to what a patient should take after surgery, especially the medications to ease any pain one might be experiencing. The same can be said for supplements. There are many supplements that boast what they can do to help with health and healing, but if you don't know how these supplements are going to react to other medications, you should avoid them.

ASPIRIN, FOR PLASTIC SURGERY, IS NOT CONDUCIVE TO EITHER RELIEVING PAIN OR FIGHTING INFECTION.

Aspirin is one of those medications that should be avoided. Aspirin is indeed a miracle drug for many different maladies; however, for plastic surgery it is certainly not conducive to either relieving pain or fighting infection. In fact, the total contrary can be said for aspirin. This drug thins the blood and could even cause excessive bleeding and slow the healing of wounds. It is better to avoid this medication and use something that will actually help to relieve the pain without the worry of other issues.

Another misconception in supplements is the application of Vitamin E, either orally or topically, to incision sites in order to help with the healing process. The confusion here comes from the idea that Vitamin E can be used in the effective improvement of scarring. Unfortunately, there is no solid evidence of this. In reality, Vitamin E has been known to cause skin irritation when applied topically and should be avoided after facial surgery. It is recommended to check with your medical team regarding the validity and function of any Vitamin supplement or medication that you want to take during your healing stage. More often than not, we will already have given you guidelines and recommendations of what medications and supplements you should take to help with your healing process.

Some of the supplements that we might have recommended to you prior to surgery should be continued for a few weeks after the healing process has begun. Often these supplements have been proven to help with wound healing, building new collagen, and decreasing inflammation and swelling. These supplements build the 'cement' that holds our cells together and allows them to thrive during the healing process.

Be certain to check with your doctor to ensure that he is in agreement, but some of the supplements that you might take to help with the healing process include:

VITAMIN A: 10,000 IU per day, beginning a week before surgery (unless you are pregnant).

VITAMIN C: 500 – 1000 mg per day, beginning a week before surgery.

ZINC: 15 mg per day, beginning a week before surgery.

ARNICA MONTANA: A natural herbal supplements that can help with bruising or soreness. It can be taken in pellet or tincture form beneath the tongue once you're awake in the recovery room.

BROMELAIN: Another homeopathic natural remedy that can help reduce bruising and swelling beginning immediately following surgery.

Again, I must reiterate that all of this should be discussed in detail with your medical team. I offer my patients a supplement healing pack that contains Arnica Montana and Bromelain as part of their aftercare and surgical healing package. You will also be given clear instructions on what medications you should continue to take after your procedure is complete and what, if any, medications should be continued even on the day of surgery.

In addition to the above supplements, I also offer my patients a Platelet Healing Gel. Platelet-rich plasma is essentially derived by drawing blood from one's arm, spinning it in a centrifuge to spin out all the platelets and healing parts of the blood, concentrating them several hundred times to what the amount normally found in the blood and tissues, and then injecting it into the areas I am treating. The goal is to help heal the skin more quickly and reduce bruising.

In most cases, there is actually very little pain medication needed for plastic surgery. In fact, many procedures require nothing more than a dose of Extra Strength Tylenol to alleviate any discomfort. As I have stated before, "The strain in pain lies mainly in the brain," can certainly be applied again here. However, I know that any pain experienced can be real pain with real discomfort, and so I take it seriously when my patients express discomfort or feeling pain. I do not hesitate to prescribe appropriate pain-relieving medicine when necessary.

MOVING **FORWARD**

We have discussed a great deal in this chapter about both the physical and mental (emotional) aspects of your facial plastic surgery recovery. Indeed, the potential for pain is real and a lot of the recovery must inherently deal with the physical and mental aspect of relieving this pain first and foremost. This is why it is so important to get relaxed, eat properly, and establish yourself back into your regular routine as slowly and smoothly as you can.

Remember at the Clevens Face and Body Specialists Center for Post-Procedural Care, we will provide you with clear and specific post-operative instructions for each particular surgery. Beyond those instructions you will also receive personal, on-going healing support and reassurance. You will be in the best of care moving forward by working with our " Image Consultant."

This person will help you through the process of caring for yourself in the post-procedural steps and advising you on how to get the best results from your own unique surgery. Our professional nurses will frequently follow up on your condition and progress, and there will be one-on-one personal visits from me. The health and welfare of my patients is extremely important. I am invested in the health, safety, and well-being of my patients going forward after surgery has been completed.

PEOPLE IN THE KNOW
PERSONAL TESTIMONIALS

b ecause post-procedural care is so important to my staff and me, we often hear from patients that the best part of the process was connected to how they were treated after the surgery itself.

Another patient, Kathryn, a 42 year old human resources manager from Satellite Beach, Florida, who opted for a Weekend Necklift, talks very highly of our post-procedural care nurses when she enthusiastically shared:

After surgery, both nurses Kendall and Toni really followed up – they just didn't send me home and forget about me. And once the surgery healed, they taught me how to take care of my skin. Actually, it's the whole team at the Clevens Center that really comes through. I am nothing but totally satisfied with the care I received during the surgery process and even now, much later. Actually, I should have done this a long time ago – without hesitation."

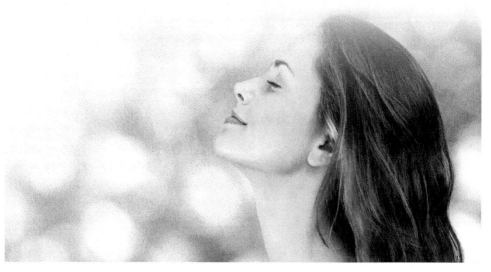

∨ BEFORE; Dan, 52 year old

∨ AFTER;Dan, 52 year old

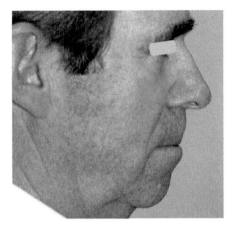

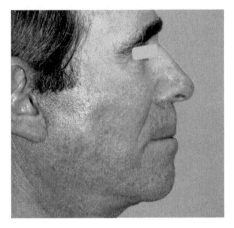

PEOPLE IN THE KNOW
PERSONAL TESTIMONIALS

Dr. Clevens performed a very successful full facelift and blepharoplasty on 55 year old patient Dan. Now Dan was a heavy smoker, but he knew that if he wanted to undergo the surgery and receive the maximum results and benefits, he would simply have to stop smoking for several weeks. Here's what he has to say about his experience:

Well, when Dr. Clevens told me I would have to stop smoking, caution lights went up all over the place. I had been smoking since I was a teenager – how was I going to quit just like that? I started out in my mind thinking that I wasn't going to smoke for only 2 weeks. But one thing led to another, and now I've been 2 years without a cigarette. I can't lie to you, every day the craving knocks on my door and I still want one. But I got to tell you, I sure feel a lot better. I can actually breathe without having to think about breathing. Plus, I don't have all that bad after-taste that can get kind of gross. Nor do I have that horrible morning cigarette breath. I'm not squinting anymore 'cause no smoke gets in my eyes – so that right there saves me a lot of wrinkles. And what's really nice is that I'm not coughing anymore, especially in the morning. What a relief! So, I truly got a double whammy here with Dr. Clevens. I got my nice facelift and bleph, looking like a million, and on top of that I feel a lot better. Why, I'd be willing to bet I added literally years to my life now that I don't smoke. The quality of life just seems a lot better now that I don't smoke. And, I got to tell you, my face? Absolutely tops! So, a new face and a better quality of life? It doesn't get any better than that! Thank you, Dr. Clevens – ten times over."

y this point you have made incredible progress. You have now completed Step Five – The Nurturing Process. What an accomplishment! Congratulations again! You did it! It's over! All your dreams, all your planning, all your efforts have finally come to fruition. But wait just another minute – it's not over yet.

There are still a couple more steps to consolidate and preserve your efforts in the process of moving forward. Now that you have recovered, do you think it's time to let go? Do you buy a new car and then never have it serviced? Do you purchase a new pair of shoes and never shine them afterwards? Do you make an important financial investment and never follow up afterwards? You have come all this way in changing your image to a newer you. Now you have to keep it that way.

The next step, "The Image Maximizer" will do just that! Now that you have gone through the surgery and have undergone the initial steps of the recovery and nurturing, it's time for you to start the process of maintaining and enhancing this incredible investment that you have made to yourself. This will help you to remain confident with your new appearance. Don't worry, you don't have to go it alone. In the next step we will be with you all the way and show you exactly how to keep your new look lasting a long time. Let's look at "The Image Maximizer."

YOUR **NOTES**

YOUR NOTES

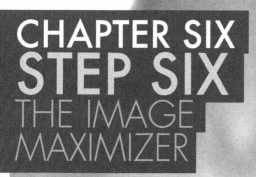

CHAPTER SIX
STEP SIX
THE IMAGE
MAXIMIZER

FROM **ONE** TO **TWELVE** MONTHS **POST** OPERATION

elcome to Chapter Six – The Image Maximizer. At this point you are well beyond that initial phase of the recovery process. You have given yourself time and space for rest, relaxation, and nurturing. You have made it through your tailor made surgical experience and you are getting back to your normal life and your typical routine. Now the focus should be placed on preserving and enhancing your surgery results. This is a very important and essential stage of the surgical process. Your new goal is to obtain the best possible, longest lasting results from the surgery itself.

This stage, which is generally from one to twelve months in duration, is where we as professionals will help you to protect your investment, which is why we call this phase The Image Maximizer. It is during this phase that we help you to take the steps that will help your look settle and last as long as possible. We will help you to stay healthy and to have healthier skin than you ever did before your surgery. It is important to us that you feel beautiful, gorgeous, confident, joyful and stay educated. Remember that there will be rather stringent rules for you to follow in order to optimize your results. Anything less may compromise your investment.

In this chapter we will discuss your diet and exercise, we will reiterate the absolute stringent rules of no smoking for at least two to four weeks after your surgery, we will go over what kind of sun exposure is acceptable, we will check in around how you are feeling, and make sure that your overall well-being is being taken into consideration. Together we will look at how you are making the all-important transition with your family, friends, and – oh yes, please do not forget about yourself.

FREQUENTLY CHECK IN AND MONITOR
HOW YOU ARE FEELING ABOUT YOURSELF

During this period we want to encourage you to frequently check in and monitor just how you are feeling about yourself. This is another point where using your surgical journal will come in handy. Keep track of your feelings around your self-assurance. Are you truly satisfied with your results? Are you gaining confidence day by day? What is your energy level like now? Are you pleased with how your surgery is settling?

How are your friends and family reacting to you at this point? Do you have any questions and concerns about your surgery going forward? It is at this stage of your process that we will start exploring the possibilities of your new skin care regimen with your personal facial skincare specialist. Our goal is to help you maintain and enhance the investment that you've made in yourself. This will also help to build and strengthen your confidence with your new appearance. Maximizing your new image is our ultimate objective at this point in time.

DIET AND EXERCISE

As far as diet and exercise is concerned, we at the Clevens Face and Body Specialists are not overly concerned with the particulars of weight control and physical training. We want you to be healthy and happy with your appearance, but we are not a weight loss and diet center. There are other centers that specialize in these types of matters. If you do have concerns about diet, health, and weight management, we can recommend places to help you. But when it comes to getting back to your eating and exercise habits from before surgery, common sense should be the norm. Your facial plastic surgery results will generally look their best if you maintain your weight around the same level as when you had your surgery performed.

We have previously mentioned that maintaining a proper diet will most certainly be beneficial to any procedure done to the face. Common sense tells us that if your face was prone to ballooning up before the surgery because of improper eating habits, then reverting back to those eating habits is going to bring the same results. By the same token, if you have been carefully monitoring your eating habits prior to the surgery, but afterwards you go on a bingeing spree, then your results and recovery could quite possibly suffer some setbacks. Gaining weight after your procedure can compromise some of the results that you have achieved.

What all of this really means is that you need to be careful with your food choices both before and after surgery. Again, common sense should reign: "Maintain consistency and everything in moderation" should be your mantra.

Over the years our common knowledge of good eating has changed dramatically. In the mid twentieth century in the United States, the traditional breakfast consisted of bacon and eggs. Now in the early 21st century we have come to find that this meal is really not so good for you after all, especially on a regular basis. In fact, this meal would probably be one of the first ones taken away from someone with high cholesterol or hardening of the arteries.

Over the years there has been a lot of research done on what foods should be eaten to help you to recover from surgeries. In the following section we have made a list of some of the things you should consider when it comes to your food intake during your recovery process.

Drink Plenty of Water. This may seem obvious, but so many patients neglect this important step for healing and long term recovery. Staying sufficiently hydrated throughout your recovery is going to help your healing process and keep your systems flushed. Recovering patients should drink at least 64 ounces of water per day.

Avoid Caffeine and Alcohol. Stay away from caffeinated beverages such as soda, tea or coffee. These types of drinks are fine in moderation. However, caffeine acts as a diuretic and can affect hydration status if someone were to drink it in excessive amounts. Sports drinks are useful only after a game! These are often high in sodium and will not replenish the body as well as water. Also, be wise about alcohol; it can in no way help to hydrate your body. Alcohol actually causes dehydration by tricking your body into losing more fluid than it gains.

Eat Nutritious Foods. This doesn't just mean foods that taste good, but foods that are good for you. Eating more fruits and vegetables than meats, starches, or sugars is common sense, and yet so many patients don't follow this simple rule. Eat healthy and you will help your body to recover sooner. A diet rich in low glycemic index foods maintains a healthy and constant blood sugar level. With high glycemic index foods, your blood glucose spikes and you become hungry quicker, consuming more calories overall. Low glycemic index foods include stone ground whole wheat, pumpernickel bread, rolled or steel cut oatmeal, oat bran, muesli, pasta, sweet potatoes, beans, nuts, most fruit, vegetables and lean meats.

Watch Your Portions. It is in your best interest to monitor your portions. This is going to help you maintain a consistent body weight during your recovery, which will help the healing process and your overall look after surgery. Most nutritionists recommend eating five to six small-portioned meals a day rather than three large ones. Of course, each person is unique. If you don't know what is best for your body and you are concerned about your food intake, you might consider working with a registered dietitian or certified nutritionist.

Don't Eat Before Bed. This is a well-known fact for a healthy lifestyle. You should stop eating at least two hours before going to bed at night. This will help your body to start the digestion process and avoid going to sleep with your stomach full of food. This idea is even more important when you are healing from a facial surgery. When your body is forced to digest during your sleep, it won't have as much energy to focus on your healing during this time.

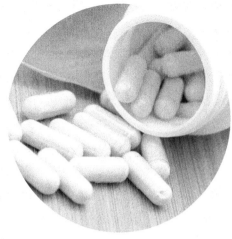

HERBS AND SUPPLEMENTS

hile in the recovery process from your facial plastic surgery, you need to be careful with the herbs and supplements that you consume. An entire list of these items has been created over the years and the details of what you personally should, and should not, be taking can be provided by your medical team.

Below you will find a list of a few herbs and supplements that could aid in your healing process. But again, don't start taking any supplements without first checking with your medical team.

Zinc   This supplement can help to reduce the healing time. It helps to boost the immune system, which can ward off infection. Zinc can be taken orally or it can be put right on the wound site with a lotion. Zinc deficiency is common, and many people can benefit from adding this supplement to their daily routine. Food sources for zinc include meat, fish, poultry, shellfish, dairy products, legumes and grains. When selecting a grain, choose whole grains whenever possible.

Vitamin C   This anti-oxidant supplement has been proven to help people heal and recuperate faster. Vitamin C is required in order for your body to create collagen. Collagen is the building block of new skin, which will help heal incision sites. Vitamin C can also help to boost the immune system and help to fight off possible infection. Food sources for vitamin C are plentiful: citrus fruits, tomatoes, both green and red peppers, cantaloupe, Barbados cherries, guava, kiwi, strawberries, brussel sprouts and more.

PHARMACEUTICAL-GRADE **SUPPLEMENTS** CAN **HELP EXPEDITE** THE **HEALING PROCESS** PARTICULARLY WITH **BRUISING, SWELLING, AND PAIN.**

Bromelain   This is an enzyme that is most commonly found in pineapples. It can help to reduce swelling and has proven to be as effective as ibuprofen in this regard, but without the side effects and liver damage that ibuprofen can cause.

Chlorella   This super food has been shown to help aid in the healing process and repair skin cells, bones, and wounds. It can also act as an immune system booster, helping your body to fight off infection.

In addition to the supplements and foods that can help you to heal, there are some things that you should avoid because they can delay the healing process or cause other complications. For example, the consumption of wine is not a good idea. Wine contains certain chemical agents that impede the efficient healing of wounds.

There are also certain over-the-counter medications that can be unfavorable for the healing process because they interfere with blood clotting. Be very careful taking many of the more common over-the-counter medications like aspirin, ibuprofen, Excedrin, Bayer products or anything that contains antihistamines. These medications thin the blood and can lead to excessive bleeding and bruising during and after your surgery. If you have any doubts about what you should, or should not, be taking you can also consult with me or anyone on your health care team.

Something that we offer our patients at the Clevens Face and Body Specialists, which can help in the area of diet, is what we call the VitalMedic Package. This package is ideal in supplying the proper nutrients that are required to maintain nutritional consistency in the body, both before and after facial plastic surgery. These pharmaceutical-grade supplements can help expedite the healing process for both surgical and non-surgical procedures. They work particularly well in helping with bruising, swelling, and pain.

The VitalMedic Package consists of a variety of pills, oils, and creams for daily consumption and application. VitalMedic is registered with the FDA and all of the ingredients are safe, quality assured, and very effective. The items in this package are geared towards specific stages of your surgery, including pre-surgical usage.

Some of the packets include the Surgery Program Packet, the Healing Supplements Program, the Anti-Aging Formula and more. Our Aesthetician and the skincare specialists in our center can outline a program tailored for your specific needs. These products can help you to produce the most effective results for your particular operation.

SMOKING

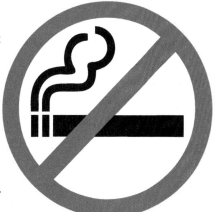

i feel compelled to make one more comment on smoking. I have addressed this issue before, but I am going to reiterate it again here. I feel that it is vitally important to refrain from smoking during the recovery period. A patient who refuses to follow his or her own pledge to refrain from smoking during their journey through the facial plastic surgery process can negate the results of their perfect surgery.

The consumption of nicotine causes the small vasculature of the skin to constrict, thereby compromising the vital blood supply to the skin and face. This can directly cause complications such as poorwound healing, increased risk of infection, longer-lasting bruises, skin necrosis, and the potential for raised and thickened scars and the increased risk of infection and respiratory complications during anesthesia.

> IF PATIENTS ARE **TAKING THE TIME, SPENDING THE MONEY, AND MAKING THE EFFORT** TO **ENHANCE THEIR APPEARANCE,** WHY WOULD THEY THEN **RISK ALL OF THAT WORK BY SMOKING?**

Our experience at The Clevens Face and Body Specialists has shown that many patients who quit smoking for four to six weeks prior to surgery remain long-term non-smokers after their surgery. We take special pride in this fact.

It is also important to reiterate that we try to encourage smoking cessation in a positive and supportive fashion.

SUN EXPOSURE

We are equally adamant about the prospect of sun exposure for our recovering patients. Exposure to the sun can be absolutely devastating to anyone's new appearance. We have briefly discussed this previously in Chapter Five, The Nurturing Process, but we feel that it is prudent to bring it up again here and strongly emphasize the importance of protecting oneself from the sun's extremely harmful ultraviolet radiation.

Indeed, the sun is no friend to recent patients of facial plastic surgery, especially when considering just how sensitive the skin is to the sun's rays. Many negative ramifications can result from a patient's exposure to the sun. This can include stimulating genetic mutations in skin cells, provoking the aging process, and inciting age spots and wrinkles. For patients who have undergone a skin resurfacing procedure, premature exposure to the sun may induce unwanted blotchiness or varying color tones in the skin.

The best way to avoid any of these problems would be to simply not go out in the sun at all. However, we understand that is impractical and, in moderation, we need sunshine to stay healthy. Twenty minutes of sun exposure is more than enough time for the average person to absorb the necessary amount of vitamin D.

FACTS ABOUT SUN EXPOSURE

Skin cancer is the most common form of cancer in the United States.
More than 3.5 million skin cancers in over two million people are diagnosed annually.
Each year there are more new cases of skin cancer than the combined incidence of cancers of the breast, prostate, lung, and colon.
Each year there are more new cases of skin cancer than the combined incidence of cancers of the breast, prostate, lung, and colon.
One in five Americans will develop skin cancer in the course of a lifetime.
Over the past 31 years, more people have had skin cancer than all other cancers combined.

Actinic keratosis is the most common pre-cancer; it affects more than 58 million Americans.
Basal cell carcinoma (BCC) is the most common form of skin cancer; an estimated 2.8 million are diagnosed annually in the US. BCCs are rarely fatal, but can be highly disfiguring if allowed to grow.
Squamous cell carcinoma (SCC) is the second most common form of skin cancer. An estimated 700,000 cases are diagnosed each year in the US, resulting in approximately 2,500 deaths.
Between 40 and 50 percent of Americans who live to age 65 will have skin cancer at least once.
About 90 percent of non-melanoma skin cancers are associated with exposure to ultraviolet (UV) radiation from the sun.
Treatment of non-melanoma skin cancers increased by nearly 77 percent between 1992 and 2006.

These statistics say nothing about how sun exposure can damage the procedures that have just been done. For healing from facial surgery it would be prudent to stay out of the sun for at least the first three weeks after surgery. This is because any exposure to the sun's rays on your new appearance may incite prolonged facial swelling and other injuries previously mentioned.

Ideally you should try to avoid the sun for up to six months after your surgery. If going outside is a must during this important healing time frame, make sure that you apply a generous amount of 30 SPF sunblock on your face without rubbing it in. Make sure that the sunscreen stays on the surface of your skin so it can literally serve as a shield against the rays. Don't forget to wear a wide-brimmed hat when you venture outside and try to stay in the shade as much as you can.

Prudence and common sense are the words to remember here. Keep in mind that your new appearance is delicate and fresh. I take great pride in the work that I have done to give you your desired results. You want to **maximize** your appearance – not **minimize** your results. I don't want anything to compromise my work or your hard-won new appearance.

CHECKING IN

s mentioned in the previous chapter, we will want to keep in contact with you during this stage, not only to monitor your physical healing, but also to monitor how you are feeling about this stage of your recovery.

There will be several visits to our center during these months where you will consult with our specialists and also with me. Together we will go through any issues, worries, or misgivings that may have come up during your healing process. Our seasoned specialists are specifically trained to handle this most important aspect of the recovery. We want you to talk to us. We are open-minded and understand your concerns.

Physically, it will be important for you to check in with yourself on a daily basis. Take some time to write down how you are feeling both emotionally and physically in your surgical journal. Have your wounds healed sufficiently to the point where you are paying less attention to them as time passes? Has your body made the appropriate adjustments to where you are now enjoying your health with a greater degree of normalcy? Has your exercise routine been producing the desired results? That is to say, is it helping to favor the results of the surgery? If so, then you should most assuredly continue with what you are doing. If not, however, then you may want to make some adjustments.

For example, if your exercise routine is causing any pain in the surgical area, then you will most definitely want to ease up and do exercises that are less stringent. If you feel your routine is too light and are not seeing the desired results fast enough, then you might consider a more aggressive workout that will create more challenges for your body. But then again, you do not want to overdo it and then cause possible risk to your wounds. The best policy here is to listen to your body and implement common sense. There is a bottom line: Are you physically feeling better?

This is also an important time to check in with how you are feeling mentally and emotionally. Remember that everyone responds to his or her surgery differently. Some people bounce right back from the operation with no mental issues whatsoever. These people are totally self-assured and absolutely positive that they did the right thing by undergoing surgery.

However, other patients do not accept their post-operative appearance very well. Are you one of those people? Do you remember the first few days when you got home after surgery? Do you remember when you looked into the mirror and saw all that swelling and all those bruises and lumps? Do you recall just how worried you were? Did you start to have second thoughts about the work you had done? Were you thrown into a depression, falsely thinking that you would always look like this and that the unsightly bruises would never go away?

These thoughts are normal and common. In fact, they occur more often than not. Nevertheless, you saw that with the passage of time, things got better. With time your wounds started to heal and your desired appearance started to emerge and blossom. Your worries and troubled thoughts started to gradually fade into a distant past and your life started to return to a more even keel of familiar activity. Your mental framework should be getting better and better by the day.

TOGETHER WE WILL GO THROUGH ANY ISSUES, WORRIES, OR MISGIVINGS THAT MAY HAVE COME UP DURING YOUR HEALING PROCESS. OUR SEASONED SPECIALISTS ARE SPECIFICALLY TRAINED TO HANDLE THIS MOST IMPORTANT ASPECT OF THE RECOVERY.

Whatever the case may be at this stage in your recovery process, your thoughts should definitely be waning from the surgery and moving on to your new projected life. You should be moving forward as a person with a new sense of self-confidence and strength.

As you move forward, it is also a good idea to check in and write about how things are going with your family and friends. Has your family helped you out during this period of transition? How much? How little? What role have they been taking in your recovery process? How important are they to you as you move forward with your new appearance? How did they receive your new look? Did they embrace it with open arms, knowing just how important the new change was for you? Or did they reject it, perhaps thinking that all this time, money and effort could have been invested in something else. After all, they are the ones that are closest to you and they are the ones that perhaps notice the biggest changes. How have their lives fared doing this whole process?

PEOPLE IN THE KNOW
PERSONAL TESTIMONIALS

If you recall, I mentioned patient Carol, who said that after her surgery her husband was a tremendous help. However, he became very overwhelmed by the ordeal and hoped that he wouldn't have to go through it again. In fact, Carol did recommend that anyone undergoing facial plastic surgery with significant post-operative downtime should unhesitatingly look into hiring a private nurse to take care of things. Subjecting one's spouse to the rigors of post-operative care can be extremely stressful and taxing.

On the other hand, remember patient Anne who underwent a facelift, an eyelid lift or blepharoplasty, and a full face laser skin resurfacing? She said that when her son saw her for the first time several weeks after the surgery, he was just taken aback at how stunningly beautiful she looked, receiving her with open arms.

As our patient Katie, a 38 year old rhinoplasty patient said when she approached this stage:

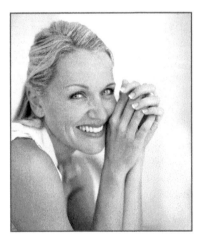

Surgery didn't really change my life as much as it changed my self-esteem and my knowledge of what this profession can do for people."

"The Clevens Center & Staff have been instrumental in my successful facial plastic surgery journey. Thank You!"

THE FAMILY AND FRIENDS REACTION

*t*he reaction of the family can truly set the foundation for a solid recovery moving into the "Maximizer" stage. But how is the family now at this stage? Whether they have accepted you with open arms or rejected your efforts wholeheartedly, has your relationship resumed a natural course of peace and harmony or has it spiraled into an area of uncertainty and discord? Whatever the case, life must move on and your family relationships should be moving into the direction of normal, loving interaction – regardless of facial plastic surgery or not!

The same thing goes with your friends. Friends can be an extremely important factor in your transition towards complete recovery as well. Sometimes, more often than your family, your friends are going to have a very strong effect on your mental state. Friends can display very powerful reactions to your new appearance. Of course, the best reactions are the ones that accept you as the way you are no matter what your appearance. However, any change does naturally provoke comments, and sometimes there can be no shortage of comments when you transition yourself back to your circle of friends.

There can be a wide variety of reactions from friends, ranging from the "Oh, I didn't notice" routine, to the highly dramatic, response of "Oh my God who beat you up? You look terrible!" Both of these extremes can put you into some serious self doubt about the choices that you have made, not to mention confusion about where your friendships might stand after these changes.

> **LIFE** MUST MOVE ON **AND YOUR FAMILY RELATIONSHIPS** SHOULD BE MOVING **INTO THE DIRECTION OF NORMAL,** LOVING INTERACTION –

Unfortunately, sometimes your friends and family members can be cruel, for whatever reason. Sometimes friends or family members will be jealous. This jealousy could be related to many things, but often it is connected to the fact that you had the initiative, the time, and the money to go ahead and actually have facial plastic surgery. They might be jealous because they don't have these resources and consequently can't get surgery themselves. Or the jealousy may come from the simple fact that you now look gorgeous. Whatever the reason, the people in your life can indeed be cruel. True friends will extend a helping hand and interact with you with love and understanding.

TIME FOR
REFLECTION

t The Image Maximizer stage it is good to put some thought and reflection on how the transition back to your friends has been. This is another time where you should take advantage of your journal. Has it been a smooth and easy transition? Where have there been rocks in the road?

The bottom line is: What about you? How are you feeling about yourself? Are you reassured now that you did the right thing? Are you satisfied with the results? Are you strong and confident? As professionals, we understand these questions may bring up concerns and this is completely normal. All patients will have some questions and concerns after undergoing facial plastic surgery. This is true even a year after the surgery.

It is for this very reason that we at the Clevens Face and Body Specialists provide consultation service for these issues. Our professionals know how to address these matters and we are truly concerned about your welfare both mentally and physically. We know how to calm, cheer, comfort, soothe, sweeten, educate, illuminate, and inspire. Remember that our philosophy at the Center of Excellence is to care for you from the beginning of the process to the end – whenever that end may be. We do not simply perform a surgical procedure and then consider the case to be closed.

On the contrary, our goal is to see you blossom into the person that you envision yourself to be, both on the outside and on the inside.

We work hard to help you gain a new version of yourself – growing into that visualization of you, gaining confidence and renewed strength each day. The "Image Maximizer" stage is the time for you to reassess yourself and your relations with those around you.

"SURGERY DIDN'T REALLY CHANGE MY LIFE AS MUCH AS IT CHANGED MY SELF-ESTEEM AND MY KNOWLEDGE OF WHAT THIS PROFESSION CAN DO FOR PEOPLE."

– *Katie Stevenson*

It is a time where you want to take stock in your new appearance and how you want to move forward. This is where you want to educate yourself about your facial skincare treatment and learn how to maintain your new image for as long as possible. After all, you have put all this time, money and effort into your new appearance; educating yourself will only bolster your efforts and empower your drive.

Indeed, you are gorgeous and you want to keep it that way. Hence, watch your diet and exercise; keep those no-smoking/no-sun exposure rules; continue to monitor your feelings about your family and friends. Make all of this an integral part of your lifestyle and you will most assuredly glow and shine like the person you have truly dreamed of becoming.

By this point you have made tremendous progress. You have now completed step six – The Image Maximizer. What an accomplishment! Congratulations again! You did it! It's over! All your dreams, all your planning, all your efforts have finally come to fruition.

Of course, just like being healthy, things aren't over yet. There is still one final step that you need to take in order to consolidate and preserve your efforts in the process of moving forward. There is one final step in the sense that this last step is really a lifelong, ongoing lifestyle process that should never end. Because of what you have been through, you are now so conscientious about facial plastic surgery and its lifetime effects both physically and mentally that you have incorporated this knowledge into your way of living. It should now become second nature.

As our patient Katie, a 38 year old rhinoplasty patient said when she approached this stage, "Surgery didn't really change my life as much as it changed my self-esteem and my knowledge of what this profession can do for people."

It is the new you that is going forward in life with this amazing sense of self-confidence. You will have all of the keys that you need to maintain your new self-image. Confidence should be part of your nature. You have come all this way in changing your image to a newer you. Now you have to keep it that way. The next step, "The Image Expander" is going to help you do just that.

You have gone through the surgery, you have taken the initial steps of healing and recovery, and now you take the most important step, maintaining and enhancing your investment and being confident in your new appearance and state of mind. We will show you precisely how to do this in our last-but not-least final step of your successful facial plastic surgery, "The Image Expander."

YOUR **NOTES**

YOUR NOTES

CHAPTER SEVEN
STEP SEVEN
THE IMAGE
EXPANDER

FROM **12** MONTHS POST OPERATION AND **BEYOND**

elcome to Chapter Seven – "The Image Expander." Wow! Now you have made it to the final step in the *A Consumer's Guide to Facial Plastic Surgery, Your Plastic Surgery Companion* You have made it through the sixth stage where the preservation of your surgery and newfound beauty became the most important factor. Enhancing your appearance for the greatest period of time and with the greatest amount of health is now your goal.

Throughout this process you have obtained the results you desired. Although the surgery, along with the accompanying process, has gradually reached closure, your new life has begun. You have addressed what bothered you and now you are moving onward, putting your (new) best face forward. Remember that during this period our central focal point has been your health and well-being, and this has played out with you feeling beautiful, attractive, confident, joyful and educated. Now that we have reached the final stage of the process, we want you to expand on this knowledge where you can go forward with confidence and without the need for constant vigil.

That is to say, you simply won't need us as much as you did before. As the great, innovative educator Maria Montessori once said, "The greatest sign of success for a teacher is to be able to say that the children are now working as if I did not exist." Well, I don't want to go so far as to say that we at the Clevens Face and Body Specialists no longer exist in your mind, rather we will always be here to help anytime you need us; but the reality is that you won't need us that much anymore.

Having been with us for quite some time now, we think that you have progressed to the point where your own knowledge will be able to lead you to exactly where you need to go. This is not to say, however, that you are on your own. We will always be here to help and guide; after all, our patients are important to us. This is true on the first day that a patient walks into our center. This is true throughout the entire surgical process: before, during and after surgery. And this is true beyond the healing process. We want you to continue your education with us. We want you to remain enlightened on the treatments and products that we offer all of our patients so that you remain informed and can continue to expand your knowledge in the field that we love.

n this final chapter, "The Image Expander," we will cover some of the non-surgical treatments that are available to enhance and expand your results. These options can help people from all walks of life enhance their facial appearance and maintain a desired image with minimal intervention by us as the professionals.

We will go over, in detail, information about injectables and fillers. We will explain just what these things can do and what their specific purposes are. We will explain exactly how they work, the duration of the treatments, and the precautions that one should take. In this chapter we will spotlight our most popular products. These are the products that our patients have found to be the most effective in enhancing and maintaining appearance. We go over the costs, the considerations, the alternatives and the future of these products. In this chapter we will explain the potential dangers of products and the precautions that must be taken.

These days, more and more people are seeking out procedures that are referred to as "injectables." These procedures work to help you obtain, and maintain, a more youthful appearance. The term 'injectable' is what plastic surgeons and skin-care specialists refer to as a 'procedure that requires the use of a hypodermic needle to perform the treatment.' In an injectable procedure, the professional will inject a serum directly into the skin of the face itself, initiating a variety of effects. The goal of these injections is for the face to take on a more youthful appearance by smoothing out the surface, by eliminating unsightly wrinkles and lines, and by filling in areas that aid in maintaining the overall conformity of the facial surface.

Before further discussion, I need to emphasize that injectables can often complement your facelift surgery, but they can never take the place of a full facelift itself. Oftentimes facelift surgery does not eliminate all wrinkles and lines, especially marionette lines and nasolabial folds. Marionette lines are the grooves that form at the corners of our mouths and extend down to the jawline and jowl. The nasolabial folds are the creases that form from the corners of our nose to the mouth. Complementary injections can help out considerably. All injectables should be done via professional consultation and professional implementation. Someone should never perform this type of procedure without specific medical and surgical training in facial plastic surgery. Today, all sorts of practitioners perform cosmetic skin enhancement, from dentists to gynecologists. Be certain that you always trust your face to a specialist who is board certified by the American Board of Facial Plastic and Reconstructive Surgery (www.abfprs.org).

ALL INJECTABLES SHOULD BE DONE VIA PROFESSIONAL IMPLEMENTATION. SOMEONE SHOULD **NEVER** PERFORM THIS TYPE OF PROCEDURE **WITHOUT** SPECIFIC **MEDICAL AND SURGICAL TRAINING IN FACIAL PLASTIC SURGERY.**

Let's move on to a discussion of the more common injectables that are applied at the Clevens Face and Body Specialists today. This information is intended for general education purposes only and should not be relied upon as a substitute for professional and/or medical advice.

THE 'RELAXERS'
BOTOX, DYSPORT AND XEOMIN

the most common and most popular injectable today is the botulinum toxin, a muscle 'relaxer.' In fact, Botox and the other relaxers, Dysport and Xeomin, have been the most popular nonsurgical cosmetic procedure performed in the United States for years now, according to the American Society of Aesthetic Plastic Surgery. In 2011, there were over 2.5 million Botox, Dysport and Xeomin procedures performed in that year alone.

Fillers and relaxers should be performed by qualified individuals. It is unfortunate that today non-plastic surgeons such as family doctors, gynecologists, anesthesiologists and even non-physicians such as dentists, oral surgeons and chiropractors are performing relaxer and filler injections. Keep in mind that, although safe, these treatments are not foolproof. Complications do occur. Saving money is great, but do you really want to save a hundred dollars and end up with a crooked face or lumpy lips? I don't know many plastic surgeons that fill cavities, but unfortunately I do know a lot of dentists who inject Botox. It is more costly to correct the errors of non-qualified and unethical practitioners than it is to do the job right in the first place.

Botox is so popular that it has become a frequent talking piece on many mainstream television shows. Talk show hosts are known to frequently poke fun at this popular cosmetic procedure. Jay Leno once quipped, "According to a new study, Botox injections can help back pain. So you see, that's why John Kerry had all that Botox – his back was killing him from all that flip-flopping on issues." Comedian Jon Stewart is also known to frequently add Botox jibes into his act. In one example he was talking to one of his correspondents, Rob Corddry.

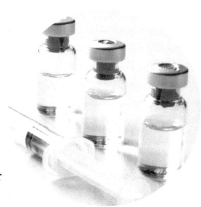

ob told the comedian that his recent Botox treatment had left him looking great, but unable to put any solids or liquids into his diet. And, of course, late night star Jimmy Kimmel got his two-cents in about Botox when he said the following: "Botox has announced that Botox can be used to tighten breasts. The only problem is your breasts always look surprised."

With all joking aside, the 'relaxers' known as Botox, Xeomin and Dysport have all been great friends to skin-care specialists because of their consistent results. It has also been a great friend for cosmetic procedure patients because it can produce almost immediate results with literally no downtime for recovery and at a relatively low cost.

THE 'RELAXERS' WORKS BY TARGETING THE MUSCLES THAT ARE THE INITIAL CAUSE OF THE WRINKLES

These 'relaxers' work by targeting the muscles that are the initial cause of the wrinkles in the first place. When the muscles are injected with the botulinum toxin, the nerve impulses that cause the wrinkles are blocked. Facial wrinkles such as frown lines and crow's feet are common target areas for this effective injectable.

The injections themselves usually cause about as much discomfort as a mosquito bite. It is also common to have a touch of bruising or swelling after Botox injections. Nevertheless, the discomfort, bruising, and swelling subside rather quickly. The results are nearly immediate withmost patients who see noticeable effects only three to five days later. And, you can return to work in most instances the same day.

An entire Botox treatment takes only five to ten minutes, but it is important to remember that the effects of this procedure are only temporary; the wrinkles do, and will, return. Relaxers work at the molecular level by binding to the muscle and blocking the action of the muscle. This temporarily weakens or paralyzes the muscle and this blockade action naturally wears off in three to six months. The muscle then returns to its normal pre-Botox state. Patients often ask if their wrinkles will be worse once the Botox wears off and the answer is no. The muscle returns to its prior state of activity once the Botox, Xeomin or Dysport wears off. You are right back to where you started. The cost for these injections will range depending on the amount of relaxer being used and the areas of the face where the injections take place. Expert injectors generally charge more because of their experience in the art of treating patients with this technique. Expect to pay more if you wan the best possible outcome and longest lasting result.

A **WORD** ABOUT **DYSPORT** AND **XEOMIN**
AS COMPARED WITH BOTOX

otox has become a household word. It is almost a generic term, like Kleenex for facial tissues. But, just like Kleenex, there are several brands of muscle relaxers. Alternatives to Botox are the FDA-approved cosmetic agents known as Dysport and Xeomin. At the time of this writing, these are the only three muscle relaxers approved in the United States by our Food and Drug Administration (FDA). By comparison, in Europe, there are literally dozens of comparable muscle relaxers on the market. Dysport and Xeomin are becoming increasingly popular for various reasons among both women and men. Although the principle of each agent works very similarly to that of Botox in that it paralyzes the muscles that cause the wrinkles, Dysport seems to work faster with longer-lasting results and Xeomin seems quite comparable to Botox in most respects.

Dysport will start to show results within just one day of application while Xeomin takes a few days to a couple of weeks for the results to become apparent. The duration of the effects for Dysport are known to last somewhat longer than the average three to six months for Botox injections. The results of Xeomin closely parallel those of Botox. The cost of the Dysport and Xeomin treatments are similar to that of Botox.

THE **HYALURONIC** **ACID** FILLERS

estylane, Perlane and Juvederm are among the most popular hyaluronic acid (HA) fillers. Whereas in the United States we have only a handful of FDA approved HA fillers, the European market has approved over 75 HA filler products. HAs are highly effective for treatment of wrinkles around the mouth and eyes. HA fillers and Radiesse (see below) can also be used to improve the nasolabial folds. Smokers' lines and vertical creases around the mouth respond nicely to Restylane and Juvederm treatments. Restylane and Juvederm also smooth crow's feet around the eyes.

WITH A JUVEDERM, RESTYLANE OR PERLANE TREATMENT THERE IS HARDLY ANY DOWNTIME AT ALL.

HA injectables can help with the contours of the lips, turned down corners of the mouth, and even the vertical furrows of the lip. Restylane, Perlane and Juvederm can be used to create a fuller looking set of lips, as well. Perlane is a bit heavier and thicker than Restylane and Juvederm. Because of this, we recommend Perlane over Juvederm or Restylane for the treatment of deeper folds where the skin is also thicker. While Perlane is too dense for crow's feet in the fine skin around the eyes, it is great for deeper nasolabial folds and marionette lines.

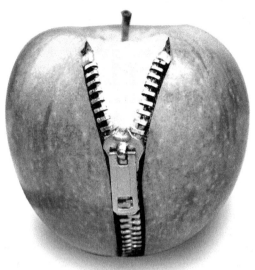

With this treatment there is a slight burning sensation during the injection. However, a desensitizing cream can be used prior to treatment. This will help to alleviate discomfort to a considerable degree. The Restylane and Juvederm injections can last anywhere between four to six months. However some patients have reported longer time effectiveness with Restylane than Juvederm. Perlane can last up to one year.

Juvederm is a newer product, manufactured by the same company that brought us Botox. This injectable has fast grown in popularity because it is very effective and easily changes the look of the face. Like the effects of Restylane, Juvederm is quite effective in adding volume under the surface of the skin. This is why it is most often used to plump up the areas around the mouth. Juvederm has been found to be especially effective in lip augmentation, marionette line reduction, and scar modification.

With a Juvederm, Restylane or Perlane treatment there is hardly any downtime at all. Although, with lip treatments, there is a certain amount of noticeable swelling that can last for several days. The cost of this treatment will vary depending on the amount of filler that is being used and the area of the injections and the expertise of the injector.

RADIESSE

Radiesse is a volumizing soft tissue filler that is FDA-approved for the correction of facial wrinkles and folds. Radiesse is thicker and more dense than most of the HA fillers and so it is best used in deeper folds such as the nasolabial folds. Most side effects of treatment resolve within a few days and, like HA fillers, many patients return to work and play immediately after treatment. Radiesse immediately provides the volume and lift needed to diminish the signs of aging because of the calcium-based microspheres and gel that comprise the product. Radiesse acts as a scaffold under the skin plumping deep wrinkles and facial folds. Experience shows that Radiesse lasts a year or more in many patients. In some ways, Radiesse is viewed as intermediate between the HA fillers (Juvederm, Restylane and Perlane) and the volumizing filler Sculptra (below). Radiesse is intermediate because it provides many of the same plumping advantages of the HA fillers while also providing the volumizing effects of Sculptra.

SCULPTRA

not only is Sculptra a newcomer on the cosmetic market, it has also revolution-ized the way we think about aging and rejuvenation. It is a 'volumizing' agent and is the only filler of its type on the US market. This product gained a significant amount of fame because it was used in the treatment of HIV. Patients who are treated for HIV lose facial fat and volume as a result of the disease and its treatment. These individuals become terribly gaunt and hollow appearing as their treatment progresses. Sculptra is highly biocompatible in HIV patients. This means that the product was very well tolerated with very few cases of allergy, rejection or unfavorable reaction. Instead, Sculptra was found to last for years with very few problems or complications in the HIV population. Over the past decade, Sculptra proved itself as a successful material especially effective in treating facial fat loss. This unique filler is now applied to the cosmetic surgery patient seeking facial rejuvenation.

Aging is often described in analogy to a beach ball. The youthful face is full, round and firm, like a fully inflated beach ball. As we age, the face loses volume and deflates like a beach ball that has lost air and has withered. This loss of volume as we age is primarily a result of losing facial fat and soft tissue. Sculptra is used to volumize or re-inflate the aging face to restore a more youthful and full appearance.

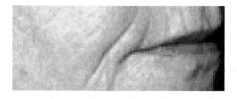   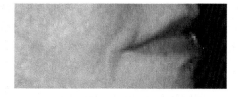

Sculptra is distinctly different from the HA fillers such as Restylane, Juvederm and Perlane. The HA fillers are best used to address individual lines and wrinkles, such as crow's feet, nasolabial folds and marionette lines. Sculptra is used as a volumizer to create a liquid facelift. Sculptra lifts the cheeks and jowls to create a more youthful facial shape. Sculptra is injected into the areas where there has been facial fat loss, resulting in a sunken, hollow, or sagging appearance in the face. This filler does not replace the fat loss, but rather, it increases the thickness of the skin in the area, thereby considerably improving the facial appearance.

Like the HAs and Radiesse, these injections can cause some pain, swelling, and bruising. Most often the discomfort disappears quickly. It can take anywhere from three to seventeen days for the effects of the injections to become visibly noticeable. There is the potential that multiple treatments will be required.

The desired outcome can last up to five years. Cost variations are dependent on the amount of product used and the areas of the face that have been injected.

OTHER INJECTABLES

here are many other types of injectables available on the market today. However, the more recent and more popular ones used in our center have been described above. Some of the other simple procedures and injectables we at the Clevens Face and Body Specialists administers include collagen injections, fat fillers, lip augmentation procedures, Radiesse, Perlane, injectable dermal fillers, and volumizers. A consultation with a licensed professional can help you determine which of these injectables might be the most appropriate for your needs.

Since there are so many injectables currently available and they are so popular, it is important to discuss the potential dangers that injectables can cause. Many have been banned from the market because they have been found to be harmful. It is necessary to take precautions in order to avoid the pitfalls that could produce lasting or permanent damage to your face. Even some of the more popular injectables that are considered safe can be harmful if not applied correctly.

One of these newer systems is the so-called "vampire injection" process. This system is also sometimes referred to as the "vampire facelift." These practices are somewhat controversial and not practiced by all plastic surgeons. These procedures have grown in popularity because of the recent cinematic crazes involving vampires. Films such as Twilight and its many sequels are prime examples. Ironically enough, though, these processes do not do anything to make you look like a vampire.

The practices get their name from the fact that the patient's own blood is used as the injectable agent. In this process the surgeon draws blood from the patient's arm and then processes the blood through centrifugal spinning, a machine that separates blood into its constituent components. This process will separate the platelet-containing plasma from the rest of the blood.

The platelet-rich plasma is then injected back into the face to fill in lines and wrinkles. The length of the procedure itself is approximately 30 minutes and the duration of the treatment can be estimated anywhere from fourteen to twenty months. However, the treatment can be deceptively costly, ranging anywhere from $1,000 to $3,000 per injection.

No matter which procedure you are considering, you should only work with a trained and licensed medical professional that has specific experience with the procedure and the injectable that interests you. Any form of amateur injection for this treatment should be avoided like the plague. It could literally cost you your life!

AMATEUR INJECTORS

nfortunately, there are many amateur injectors out there. These people are posing as professionals, but they are not. These charlatans will throw "Botox Parties." These so-called professionals will come to your home and inject you and your friends for one low cost. The reality is that these injectors can pose a very serious threat to the well-being of your face and to your overall health and welfare.

Deciding to get any of the injectables mentioned in this chapter requires a qualified, skilled, and experienced specialist. All of the injectables require precise knowledge of the anatomy of the face. They also require the specific knowledge of correct dosages that should be used. An unskilled, inadequately trained clinician would simply not have this knowledge and this is very dangerous.

> THESE **INJECTORS** CAN **POSE** A VERY **SERIOUS** **THREAT** TO THE **WELL-BEING** OF **YOUR FACE** AND TO YOUR **OVERALL** **HEALTH** AND **WELFARE.**

The potential side effects from any improper technique can cause severe damage not only to the face, but also internally, such as problems with swallowing or even respiratory malfunctions. Many amateurs often neglect to consider the medical history of the patient, thereby injecting the person with a total unawareness of any potentially negative reaction.

This is another one of the many reasons that these so-called popular "Botox Parties" can be so dangerous. Botox administered at private parties, in less-than-sterile conditions, by unskilled and unlicensed injectors, can be a recipe for disaster. This is why our center heavily frowns upon such parties and why we allow only trained professionals to administer any injectable in a sterile environment.

Another serious danger stemming from these types of parties is the potential for receiving a tainted or diluted agent from an unqualified individual. Some dubious practitioners use tainted agents in direct efforts to save money on their supplies or to reduce the duration of injectables. They do this to try to make more money from you by forcing you to get more frequent sessions.

In 2004, four people became paralyzed after receiving fake Botox injections at a non-plastic surgery general medical clinic in South Florida. The doctor who injected the toxin had passed off a research toxin not even approved for human use as 'real' Botox. The FDA and the US Government investigated this travesty and arrested 31 unscrupulous individuals who purposely injected an unapproved, cheaper substitute toxin for FDA-approved Botox Cosmetic into nearly 1,000 unknowing patients. A similar series of events occurred in the State of New York in 2009. Stories such as these highlight the importance of having your cosmetic facial injections performed by a qualified practitioner such as a board certified facial plastic surgeon and not just any doctor or caregiver who offers the best price.

Some reports have even revealed that non-professionals are not even using the desired agent itself. Instead, other less expensive agents such as liquid silicone or even baby oil are unwittingly being injected into the body. This is alarming, and it can produce catastrophic results. From a professional point of view, it is very hard for me to understand why anyone would ever want to take such a risk and resort to someone other than a trained professional in an appropriate environment. My philosophy on this has always been and will always remain that amateur injectors produce amateur results – Period! This is your face you are dealing with here. I would advise you to avoid amateur injectors like the plague!

If you are interested in injectables, you don't have to look any further than a Center of Excellence excellence specializing in facial plastic surgery such as Clevens Face and Body Specialists. At a center such as ours, you are assured the comfort and safety of a board certified facial plastic surgeon who has dedicated his practice to excellence. Facial plastic surgeons are individuals who have focused their career on plastic and reconstructive surgery of the face, nose, eyelids, head and neck rather then plastic surgery of the body in general and are board certified by the American Board of Facial Plastic Surgery.

 Visit www.abfprs.org or www.aafprs.org to find a facial plastic surgery specialist near you.

LASER SERVICES

here is also a lot more that we can help you with at the Clevens Face and Body Specialists. One area we pride ourselves on is offering the most modern laser services for the treatment of many different kinds of skin issues such as acne.

Many people are under the false assumption that acne is something that only adolescents have to deal with. The reality is that acne is a persistent problem with people of all ages. In fact, according to the American Academy of Dermatology (www.aad.org), acne is the most common skin problem in the United States today. Over 80 percent of people in their 20's and 30's are dealing with acne-related issues.

Smooth and clear skin is something that everyone wants to have. Women used to go out of their way to protect their clear complexion, but now we live lifestyles where it isn't possible to avoid being out in the sun. When the skin is exposed to the elements, it will age much more quickly and become damaged much more quickly, as well.

With the application of the laser, or with a non-laser alternative approach, the "Pulsed Light Acne Treatment," positive results for getting clear skin can be reached. The changes you can get from these treatments are long lasting and there are no drug-related side effects to worry about.

Laser treatment can also work wonders for patients suffering from annoying skin complications like uneven pigmentation on the face or common rosacea. Age spots, dark circles, and scars can also be considerably reduced by laser treatment. Our state of the art equipment and our trained professionals all serve to create the perfect environment to address these issues.

LASER TREATMENT CAN ALSO WORK WONDERS FOR PATIENTS SUFFERING FROM ANNOYING SKIN PROBLEMS.

After getting the laser treatment procedure, it will be important to keep your skin as moist as possible. To accomplish this, you will be given detailed instructions on how to care for your skin. To get the best results it is important that you follow these instructions explicitly. It will be vital for you to keep the crusting of the skin to a minimum. You might also need to keep a spray for your face, which will keep potential pain and discomfort down.

∨ Rosacea   ∨ Port Wine Stains   ∨ Lentigines   ∨ Telangiectases

 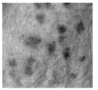 

The skin resurfacing options won't work on all skin issues that you might have. Some of the more common skin blemishes that can sometimes be treated by laser resurfacing treatments are discussed below.

Hemangiomas These blemishes are red and lumpy and are often referred to as 'strawberry marks.' They are actually the first stages of benign tumors of the blood vessels. Most often they are present at birth and fade over time. In most instances, they disappear completely.

Syringomas These blemishes develop around the eyes and along both sides of the nose. They are just simple growths that are skin colored.

Port Wine Stains These are smooth red brown stains on the skin cause by enlarged blood vessels under the skin. They appear at birth and often continue to grow through life.

Cafe Au Lait Spots Smooth and light brown in color, these birthmarks develop at birth and are caused from excess melanin. They tend to stay the same size and shape.

Dermatosis Papulosa Nigra These blemishes are only found in African-Americans and individuals of Asian descent. They are small, round, brown bumps that develop along the cheeks and near the eyes.

Xanthelasma This type of blemish grows on the eyelids. It is raised and yellow in color.

Actinic Keratoses Most often found on fair-skinned individuals, these are raised and rough patches of skin that often develop after sun exposure.

Lentigines These blemishes are also called age spots, liver spots, or freckles. They show up in older people and are often caused by sun exposure.

Seborrheic Keratoses These blemishes are warty-like thickenings of the skin that tend to form later in life.

Rosacea A skin condition that causes small red bumps to develop on the face.

Rhinophyma This is also referred to as 'red nose syndrome.' It is a type of rosacea that is only on the nose. The skin on the nose will also thicken with.

Telangiectases Also called spider veins, and are small, threadlike blood vessels that develop under the skin and look like spider webbing.

AESTHETICIAN
SERVICES

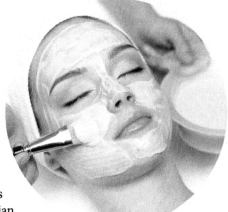

m any facial plastic surgery clinics such as Clevens Face and Body Specialists offer an array of specialized aesthetician services to help polish and maintain your image. Our practice, for example provides services in medical aesthetics, custom blended makeup, permanent makeup and waxing. Some of our aestheticians are Master Makeup Artists while others perform rejuvenative skin care such as deep pore cleansing, custom facials, medical grade peels, microdermabrasion and laser skin treatments.

Perhaps most importantly, an experienced medical aesthetician assists with the development of a proper skin care regimen. There are so many skin care products on the market. The global skin care market is almost six billion dollars. This is a truly staggering amount of money and a dizzying volume of products. A qualified aesthetician under physician supervision should be able to help you sort through the available array. Exciting and effective non-surgical services for anti-aging and skin tightening have emerged in the last few years. These technological advances include new energy delivery methods that are based on ultrasound and radiofrequency. The latest non-surgical procedures preserve the results of surgery that has been performed and can be used on their own in patients that are either contemplating or are perhaps not yet ready for surgery. Either way, a facial plastic surgery center of excellence should feature a full armamentarium of non-surgical options for patients that want minimally invasive and 'lunchtime' treatments to combat aging.

In addition to specialty services, medical aestheticians are often integrated into the after care of surgical patients. A skilled aesthetician can help a post-surgical patient with cover-up or camouflage makeup to cover bruising and swelling so that you may return to work and your usual activities more quickly. Certain aestheticians also perform lymphatic massage. Lymphatic massage is a technique performed either with a specialized machine or with the aesthetician's own hands that encourages lymph flow in the body. A healthy flow of lymph supports the body's immune system in fighting toxins and infection. Lymphatic massage also helps bruising and swelling resolve more quickly.

At first glance it might seem like the list of aesthetic services is provided mostly for women. It is true that most of our patients are women. In fact, many of them are on our program of life-long services following the Image Expander concept. However, more men are coming into our center requesting services for a variety of facial plastic surgery procedures and treatments.

THE IMAGINE MEDISPA
AT CLEVENS FACE
AND BODY SPECIALISTS

the Imagine Medispa at Clevens Face and Body Specialists offers a myriad of services that complement the desires of the facial plastic surgery patient. **Botox, Juvederm and other injectables are very popular at this clinic as well as the Aesthetician services such as chemical peels, microdermabrasion, and deep pore cleansing laser surgery.** Laser surgery is used for the treatment of such conditions as acne, rosacea, unwanted hair and scarring. This small, "mini-clinic," so-to-speak, is dedicated to high professionalism as well as the full intent of making patients happy and satisfied.

Rose is one such patient as she relates her experience with a chemical peel treatment.

" *At first I was a little reluctant to do this treatment, but after talking to the Physician Assistant to Dr. Clevens, I was convinced that my facial skin really needed to be smoothed out. Before she applied the lotion to my face she explained that the process basically cleans the skin with a combination of alcohol and acetone, and that the smell would be somewhat disagreeable. Well, I'm glad she warned me of this, because the smell was absolutely horrific. The emollients on my face tingled a little bit, and afterwards I felt a little weird for about a day or so. And then my face started peeling. I couldn't believe how much skin on my face just peeled off. But afterwards my facial skin felt baby-smooth. I love the results of this treatment. My entire face is much softer, the texture of the skin has improved tremendously and now it even has a type of glow to it. I've recommended this treatment to several of my friends already. The service is great here: friendly, understanding, caring and efficient. I didn't even have to wait. Now that's what I call service! Fantastic!"*

COSMETIC SURGERY FOR MEN

ndeed, I have been noticing over the recent years a growing trend in the number of men that are seeking out cosmetic surgery. It seems that competition in today's youth-oriented world markets is fueling men looking to increase their chances for success. As their need to compete effectively rises, so does the acceptance of cosmetic improvement among professional men.

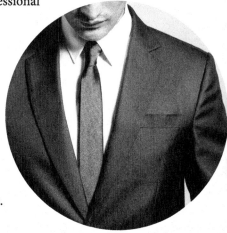

Men, just like women, have to fight against the aging process. They are starting to recognize that a more youthful appearance can be a big benefit for business. Many men seek facial rejuvenation procedures like facelifts, eyelid surgery, nose reshaping, and skin resurfacing with lasers and peels. Men are starting to feel that the reflection they see in the mirror is just as important as it has always been for women. In our society, all individuals, male or female, are appearance-conscious.

Even with these changes, many men are reluctant to explore plastic surgery options, thinking it may not be the "masculine" thing to do.

Overall it seems that most men are more amiable to plastic surgery when there are shorter healing times required. In general, men are quicker to heal and are able to return to their normal lives faster than the average woman. This makes being away from their lives much easier because it is often for a shorter amount of time.

MEN, JUST LIKE WOMEN, HAVE TO FIGHT AGAINST THE AGING PROCESS. THEY ARE STARTING TO RECOGNIZE THAT A MORE YOUTHFUL APPEARANCE CAN BE A BIG BENEFIT FOR BUSINESS.

∨ BEFORE; Actual Weekend Necklift Patient

∨ AFTER; Actual Weekend Necklift Patient

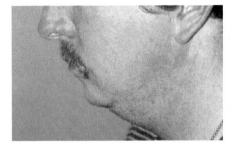

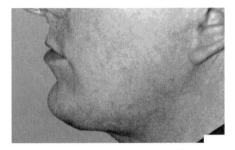

∨ BEFORE; Actual Eyelid Lift Patient

∨ AFTER; Actual Eyelid Lift Patient

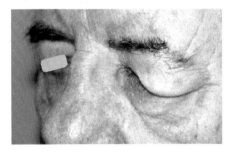

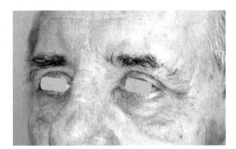

In addition, men are faced with unique considerations when contemplating cosmetic procedures. The anatomy of a man is quite different from that of a woman. A man's muscles tend to be thicker, chemical reactions in their body's are different, and a greater variance in exposed skin areas may all need to be taken into consideration. While these differences do not necessarily pose a greater possibility of complications, gender differences could be a reason for surgeons to alter procedure choice or the extent of the procedure.

Men must also take into account their tolerance for scarring and how their own body tends to heal. More often than not, men are not able to cover their scars in the facial area as well as women are able to. Hairstyle and makeup work in a woman's favor. Men are also typically much more concerned about privacy than women. They may find that they want to take more time off from work than a female counterpart because they want to make sure that any tell-tale signs of cosmetic surgery have long healed.

In my practice, one of the most popular procedures chosen by male patients is the laser assisted "weekend necklift." This surgical procedure represents the evolution of several sophisticated facial plastic surgery techniques. By combining surgical and laser techniques, I achieve improvement in the contour of the chin and neck with minimal incisions, and a rapid recovery time frame.

The first step of the weekend necklift is cervicofacial liposculpture or liposuction of the chin and neck. This is done first in order to contour the unfavorable fatty changes that can be seen in the face and neck from the passage of time. This extra skin around the neck and face is often referred to as "turkey neck" or a "double chin."

After the fatty tissues have been removed, careful attention is then turned to tightening the neck muscles and eliminating the neck bands. There is a muscle that spans our neck known as the platysma muscle. As we age, this muscle droops in the front of the neck underneath the chin. This drooping is responsible for the bands and cords that form in our necks as time passes. The last step of this process uses the laser to "resurface" the underside of the neck skin, thereby "shrink wrapping" the skin of the neck, restoring a youthful contour.

A neck lift removes excess fat and muscle in the jaw or chin area. When it comes to men getting this procedure, the beard length and side burns may be factors in deciding the appropriate place for incisions. Another consideration point for men is that a man's neck muscles are thicker than a woman's. This does not necessarily present a surgical problem or imply that there will be additional complications. Yet, it may change the extent of the procedure. The texture of a man's chin and neck skin is coarser than a woman's. This can help to reduce the appearance of scars, while beard and side burns can also cover scars.

The ultimate goal for men seeking plastic surgery is to project on the outside what they still maintain on the inside: a youthful, vibrant contributor to today's society. Men want the confidence to compete with their younger counterparts and many patients are amazed at what just a nip and a tuck can do within a very short time. For most men, the laser assisted weekend necklift procedure offers maximum cosmetic benefits with minimum downtime.

In the future, I expect to see more men coming into the center, not only to seek surgical procedures and non-surgical treatments, but also to take advantage of our Image Expander programs.

For several years now, our center has been conducting seminars for men in an effort to shed light on a subject that has traditionally been reserved for women. Hopefully, our educational endeavors will pay high dividends for both the female and male populations in our community.

THE **END** OF THE **ROAD**

his brings us to the end of step seven – The Image Expander. The thousand miles that have been part of your cosmetic journey is over. What an accomplishment! You did it! It's over! All your dreams, all your planning, all your efforts have finally come to fruition. By now you have realized that this final step is not really final at all; you have embarked on a lifestyle process that should never end.

At this point you should now be so conscientious about facial plastic surgery and its lifetime effects both physically and mentally that you have incorporated this knowledge into your way of living. At this phase, it is going to be second nature. Indeed, you have come a long way. You started out by not knowing for sure what you even wanted; but through curiosity, investigation, inquiry, and research, you took that first step into our center and into the world of facial plastic surgery. You began your journey with the one-on-one meeting with our Patient Concierge who then led you to the confidential conversation with me, Dr. Clevens.

With this Specialist Advantage, we walked you through an aesthetic game plan where we discussed, at length, your facial concerns, your before and after pictures, and the securing of your aesthetic dreams. You then prepared for the big day by moving on to the third step of making preparations and plodding through the Reassurance Program, reviewing your personal health history, filling out all the paperwork and finalizing your financial investment.

Then, the big day arrived when the surgery actually took place. You came to our center and checked in at our ambulatory surgical center. You met with your surgical nurse who was with you throughout the entire operation. You talked with the anesthesiologist and finally with me to go over last minute concerns. You went through the surgery – you endured. From there you were wheeled into recovery, stayed for a couple of hours, and then you were taken home to start your convalescence.

But the journey wasn't over, was it? You then traveled through a rather delicate period called the Nurturing Process where our professionals were always on call for you, night and day, answering your questions and making follow-up appointments.

From there, you entered the realm of the Image Maximizer where you learned about maintaining and enhancing your investment with confidence and strength. And, finally, you ended your great odyssey here with the seventh and final step, the Image Expander – only to find that it's not a final step at all, but a true launch into a lifestyle of health and well-being. As your doctor, as your teacher, and as your friend, I would like to thank you for allowing me to accompany you on your sojourn of the Seven Steps of your Facial Plastic Surgery. I wish you all the best in the continuation of your journey forward and hope that we meet again soon. ■

PEOPLE IN THE KNOW
PERSONAL TESTIMONIALS

Beverly is typical of a medispa client.

The first time I went to the Imagine Medispa, I really didn't know what to expect, because it was the first time I had ever been in contact with plastic surgery people. I did know that I wanted to smooth out the wrinkles on my face for a start, and then see what I could do for my hideous-looking turkey-neck that I had hanging underneath my chin. I was cordially received by the people at the Imagine Medispa and hardly had to wait at all. Before I knew it, I was in Lynn's room explaining to her my concerns. Lynn was so friendly and upbeat, I got along with her right away. She ended up giving me a series of Botox injections that cleared up my face right away – I couldn't believe the change happened so fast – just in a matter of hours I could see a dramatic difference – I thought it would take a couple of days, at least. Lynn recommended that I see Dr. Clevens for my depressing turkey neck, so I made an appointment right away. The following week I walked into the Clevens Center and first talked to Tanya. She told me what I needed and took computer pictures to explain to me the details. When I talked to Dr. Clevens, I was so happy to hear what he could do for me. I finally could get rid of something that had been bothering me ever since my mid-twenties. The operation went very smoothly with hardly any pain at all. That's amazing! I was surprised how well the surgery went and my recovery time was unexpectedly short. If I had known the procedure was that easy, I would have done this years ago. With my new Botox image and my new neck, I feel really beautiful and very happy. My friends even say that I have a certain glow now and my self-confidence comes out. My surgery was life-changing. I just can't help but keep smiling!"

YOUR **NOTES**

_____

_____

_____

_____

_____

_____

_____

_____

_____

_____

_____

_____

_____

_____

_____

_____

_____

_____

YOUR NOTES

CHAPTER EIGHT
A PATIENT'S GUIDE TO THE MOST COMMON FACIAL PLASTIC SURGERY PROCEDURES

his final chapter is not another step in the Seven Steps, rather, this is a guide to provide you with more detailed information concerning the most common facial plastic surgery procedures. This information is intended for general education purposes only and should not be relied upon as a substitute for professional and/or medical advice.

The procedures included in this segment are explained and detailed information is provided to help you understand more about each procedure. We go over how the surgery is actually performed, the approximate length of the operation, the projected results, the estimated recovery time and what you should consider as you contemplate your journey through your facial plastic surgery experience. The knowledge provided here will hopefully shed light and understanding on procedures that our community has found to be the most enticing to consider.

PLATELET HEALING GEL™
MINIMIZES YOUR DOWNTIME

latelet Healing Gel™ is an important technology that may help improve your results after facial plastic surgery. Clevens Face and Body Specialists innovated the use of the patient's own natural regenerative factors to speed healing and minimize downtime. Platelet Rich Plasma (PRP) has been used for years in dentistry, orthopedics, and sports medicine to assist wound healing. The Clevens Face and Body Specialists proudly pioneered the use of PRP in facial plastic surgery. Since 2001, Dr. Clevens has improved aesthetic results for over 5,000 patients with autologous unipotent stem cell technology.

Platelet Healing Gel™ or Platelet Rich Plasma (PRP) is based on the patient's natural regenerating factors to promote new tissue growth that reverses aging. The application of Platelet Healing Gel™ is performed in conjunction with certain facial plastic surgical procedures to improve your outcome, shorten your downtime and minimize bruising. Research has shown that a patient's own platelet rich plasma is a safe and cost effective way to enhance your facial plastic surgical procedure through harnessing the healing and regenerative potential of the human body to rejuvenate itself.

Platelet Healing Gel™ is a safe and rapid preparation of a soft tissue regenerator referred to as PRP. PRP is injected into the treatment area to stimulate cells, contour the face and promote an increase of volume and rejuvenation and supercharge healing. A small volume of blood is drawn from the patient and then centrifuged to separate platelets, serum and fibrin, the elements that travel in our blood and are responsible for healing. This natural solution from your own body is then activated at the time of your procedure, resulting in Platelet Healing Gel™ that promotes facial rejuvenation.

Upon administration, platelets release natural tissue regenerating factors; studies showed that platelet growth factors are released for up to seven days, supporting collagen production and dermal matrix reconstruction. Since the procedure uses no synthetic materials, there is virtually no risk of allergic reaction, and no significant adverse events have been reported. For this reason, PRP Rejuvenation Therapy can be used to enhance results in many areas to achieve facial and skin rejuvenation.

CONSIDERING
BLEPHAROPLASTY
OR EYELID
SURGERY?

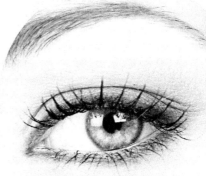

he eyes are the first place on the face that will show the signs of aging. The eyes are most certainly the focal point of the face and an increased laxity of skin can come across to others as looking tired, sad, or melancholy, even if this isn't an accurate image of how you are feeling.

Blepharoplasty surgery, or the eyelid tuck as it is sometimes called, is the surgical procedure that gives your eyes a more rested appearance. It does this by reducing the excess skin and fatty tissue that can develop in both the upper and lower eyelids with aging.

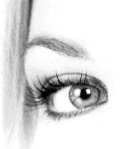

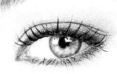

ANATOMY

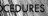

he entire eyeball is surrounded by fatty tissue, which is medically called adipose tissue. A thin membrane called the orbital septum is what holds this fatty tissue into position. With aging, the fatty tissue can bulge forward, especially in the lower eyelid. This can form a hernia, just like in any other part of the body.

The dark circles that people complain about are many times due to changes in skin pigmentation, but are also usually, at least in part, due to a shadow effect that is caused by this excess fatty tissue. The result is a bagginess or bulging of the lower eyelid that causes this shadowing effect. This is why the condition can appear worse in different kinds of light.

The appearance of dark circles can worsen during a woman's menstrual cycle. They can also seem worse when you have been eating or drinking an increased amount of sodium. Both the female menstrual cycle and increased amounts of sodium can cause an increase of fluid retention in the body. The fatty tissue attracts this fluid, which results in an increase in bulging under the eye.

If the condition is detected early, the fatty tissue can be removed simply by using a laser on the interior part of the lower eyelid. This laser process can remove the fat without any external incision. This process is called a transconjunctival blepharoplasty where an incision is made inside of the eyelid itself to gain access to the lower eyelid fat bags. The fatty tissue is removed and the skin is re-draped into its normal position.

However, if the condition has persisted for too long or if the skin laxity has markedly increased, then both skin and fatty tissue will need to be removed. This would be the traditional blepharoplasty or eyelid tuck.
The appearance of our eyes is an individual characteristic. The individual look of

our eyes is partly due to the shape of the bone cavity, also referred to as the orbit. Some people have a very prominent superior orbital rim and this will affect the shape of the overall eye area. Little can be done to alter bone structure of this area.

In some cases the depth of our eyelid crease is determined by the amount of cartilage in the eyelid area. This is an inherited characteristic and there is a limit as to how much it can be modified. For example, an individual with a smaller amount of skin on the eyelids may be able to obtain significant improvement in the appearance of his or her eyes with surgery, but surgery might not be able to change the eyelid fold due to anatomy.

FOR WOMEN, A GOOD TIME TO SEEK OUT EYELID COSMETIC PROCEDURES IS WHEN IT BECOMES DIFFICULT TO APPLY EYE SHADOW ON THE UPPER EYELID.

The signs of aging in the eyes will be noticeable for different people at different times and ages. The average person will start to lose laxity in his or her upper eyelid as early as age 25. From 25 to 30 aging will start to show on the lower eyelid as well. However, since our individual anatomy in this area varies so greatly, there are two general principles that guide the decision on when it is a good time to seek out eyelid surgery.

For women, a good time to seek out eyelid cosmetic procedures is when it becomes difficult to apply eye shadow on the upper eyelid. This is a clear sign that surgery might help you look more youthful. For men and women both, eyelid surgery might help when a good night's sleep doesn't get rid of puffiness in the lower eyelids.

Most often a droopy eyelid happens due to laxity in upper eyelid skin. Infrequently, it could be related to an abnormality in one of the upper eyelid muscles. There is a small muscle in the eye, called the levator musculature and its associated aponeurosis, which are layers of flat broad tendons. These layers can sometimes lose their attachment to the cartilage in the eyelid or can become dysfunctional with age. This can cause the eyelid to drop. This usually occurs unilaterally, although from time to time we will see this droopiness, or ptosis, in both eyes.

When this happens the muscle will need to be tightened, and any excess skin and fatty tissue in the upper eyelid area will need to be removed. When this condition occurs, there can be significant improvement, but there will always be some asymmetry or slight difference in the position of both eyelids.

SURGICAL PROCEDURE

yelid surgery is usually performed under twilight anesthesia and on an outpatient basis. In the upper eyelids a special marking pencil is used to make marks on the upper eyelid crease. Calipers are used to engage the amount of excess skin contained in the upper eyelid. This is called the 'pinch technique.'

The skin is then removed and the excess fatty tissue from the middle of the eyelid is also removed. In some cases the upper eyelid muscle may be contoured as well. The incision is closed with dissolvable sutures and/or sutures that run underneath the skin and can be painlessly removed after one week. Within approximately one week, the incision conforms to the natural contour of the eye and is hidden in the eyelid fold. Laterally, it blends in to the fine eyelid creases in the outer part of the eye.

In the lower eyelid an incision is made several millimeters below the eyelash line and is carried laterally into the skin crease. The skin and muscles are reflected down and three fatty tissue pockets in the lower eyelid are opened and excess fatty tissue is removed. The skin and muscle are then repositioned and excess skin is removed.

The incisions are closed with interrupted dissolvable sutures. Frequently special tape is used to support the lower eyelid area for a week after surgery. This helps to reduce the amount of swelling and bruising and allows an increased amount of extra skin to be removed more safely.

If the only problem in the lower eyelids is removing excess fatty tissue, this can often be done with a laser and no external incision is needed. In this case, the laser will remove the fatty tissue from inside the eyelid with no incision on the outside of the eyelid. If, however, excess fatty tissue has resulted in stretching of the lower eyelid skin, then both fatty tissue and skin will need to be removed. This requires the traditional blepharoplasty with an external incision.

MOST OFTEN WE FIND THAT WHETHER THEY HAVE **SURGERY** DONE **AT AGE 30, OR AT AGE 50, RARELY DOES THIS PROCEDURE NEED TO BE REPEATED.**

Patients commonly ask how long eyelid surgery will last. Because tissue is being removed, one will always look better than they would have had they not had the surgery. The reality is that we will continue to age and therefore, there will always be changes and aging in this area. We are fortunate that eyelid changes do not occur as rapidly after surgery as changes in other areas might.

Some individuals may require repeat surgery, but most often we find that whether they have surgery done at age 30, or at age 50, rarely does this procedure need to be repeated. This seems to be connected to the fact that the fatty tissue does not recur. Plus, the eye is located within the bony structure and appears to be protected somewhat by the gravitational and environmental effects of aging as contrasted with what happens with the cheeks, jowls, and neck area. These areas might need a follow-up procedure after a complete facelift.

Various types of chemical peels can be used to remove wrinkling in the eyelid area and provide an additional tightening effect to the skin. Chemical peels can be performed three to four months after an eyelid surgery has been completed. There are a wide variety of chemical peels that can be used. Each type of peel varies in the degree of wrinkle removal and tightening that is obtained. A new development has been the use of laser abrasions to resurface or rejuvenate eyelid skin.

RECOVERY

After an eyelid surgery, an individual should try to sleep with his or her head elevated for the first 48-72 hours. It is also important to refrain from lifting anything heavier than five pounds or participate in activities that result in heart rate elevation for the first seven to ten days following surgery. This will help to minimize the amount of swelling and bruising that will happen.

Eyelid incisions are most often cleansed with hydrogen peroxide soaked Q-tips. This should be done three to four times a day during the first week following the procedure. After 24 hours it is likely that the individual will be allowed to shower, as long as the shower spray does not directly hit the face. Depending on your healing process, this might be encouraged in order to accelerate the wound healing.

Most often makeup can be applied after seven days and this is also true of using facial cleansers and other cosmetic facial products. Applying makeup sooner could result in irritation to the incision lines and should be avoided.

Ice water-soaked compresses should be applied to the eyelid area every hour for a minimum of ten minutes for at least the first two to three days following this surgical procedure. This is a critical step towards helping to reduce swelling and bruising. Icing the area can also decrease discomfort and accelerate any wound healing. Ice packs work well, but they don't contour into all areas of the eyelid. One way to help eliminate this problem is to use a washcloth soaked in ice water or even use a bag of frozen peas.

For at least two days after surgery, eyelid movement should be kept at a minimum: This means keeping the eyes closed as much as possible and using the cold compresses. If you attempted to read, watch television, or do heavy paperwork immediately after your surgery this would be an unnecessary strain on the eyes. Plus, every time you blink there would be pulling and stretching on the incision lines, so it is better to just rest the eyes as much as you possibly can.

The more you can rest your eyes, the more you will notice a decrease in swelling and bruising. For the first 48 hours patients should have as much eye rest as possible. We would recommend listening to books on tapes, CDs, or listening to the television (but not watching).

Approximately 90 percent of patients find that, at the end of the first week, they can resume their normal activities. In ten percent of cases there may be some increased swelling and bruising; but even this can usually be camouflaged with makeup.

When lower eyelid rejuvenation and surgery is performed from inside the eyelid without a scar in the skin, a procedure known as transconjunctival blepharoplasty, patients can often return to normal social and work activities within just a few days. Advances in laser technology allow this surgery to be performed with much less discomfort, bruising, and swelling. However, this procedure can only be done if there is good elasticity to the lower eyelid skin.

CONSIDERING THE LASER ASSISTED
WEEKEND NECKLIFT™?

he Laser Assisted Weekend Necklift™ is an exciting new way to improve the look of your neck and jowl regions. This innovative procedure represents the unique marriage of three advanced techniques in facial plastic surgery: liposculpture, neck lifting, and laser resurfacing.

In The Laser Assisted Weekend Necklift™ procedure, there is only a small incision that is made under the chin and a tiny incision behind each of the ears. To restore a more youthful look to the neck and jaw line, liposuction is performed to remove any excess fat. After the liposculpture technique is performed, there is a surgical lifting and gentle tightening of the underlying muscle tissues of the neck. The last step is the laser rejuvenation technology, which is one of the most cutting edge procedures available.

Unlike some of the laser skin resurfacing procedures, the laser isn't used on the surface of the skin, but rather the laser is applied to the undersurface of the neck and jowl skin. The energy emitted by the laser actually shrinks the excess tissues and skin of the neck to restore taut jaw and neckline. This is often called the 'shrink wrap' method, and it replaces the need to cut away or remove any of the excess or sagging facial tissues.

Due to the innovative use of the laser, your skin will not have the typical sunburned appearance that is so common from the conventional laser skin resurfacing process. The Laser Assisted Weekend Necklift™ also avoids the extensive incisions that are made around the hairline and ears during a conventional facelift. Recovery time is shorter and the process is simpler in comparison to a conventional facelift surgery.

Another bonus to the The Laser Assisted Weekend Necklift™is that the procedure typically takes only about an hour-and-a-half to complete. It is done as an outpatient, same-day surgery in one of the Clevens Face and Body Specialists' accredited and licensed ambulatory surgical facilities. The procedure is done with the help of a board-certified physician anesthesiologist. This is to ensure your comfort and safety during the procedure. Unlike a traditional facelift, which needs several weeks for recovery, most patients who receive the 'Weekend Necklift' are able to resume their usual activities in less than one week.

CONSIDERING
ENDOSCOPIC FACIAL
SURGERY?

ndoscopic facial surgery is an exciting new technique that can help address laxity in the forehead, face, and neck. This procedure utilizes specially developed lasers and small telescopes that are called endoscopes. The procedure is done by operating through tiny incisions that are hidden within the hairline. The underlying fat, tendons, and muscles are precisely lifted to create a more youthful facial appearance.

Endoscopic lifting procedures are less invasive than routine full facial plastic surgery procedures. Most people experience minimal swelling and bruising and can usually return to work within a few days. Some of the specific types of 'endoscopic' facial procedures offered are summarized below:

Endoscopic Brow Lifting is performed through two tiny `keyhole' incisions placed right behind the front of the hairline. The forehead area is then elevated and repositioned. This process creates a more youthful appearance to the brow and upper eyelid region. This procedure is especially helpful in addressing specific areas of concern, such as: sagging in the eyebrow area, softening vertical lines between the eyebrows and the horizontal creases in the forehead. The procedure is also used to help contour muscles in those individuals who have severe wrinkling from excessive muscle movement in the mid-forehead region.

Endoscopic Forehead 'Muscleplasty' is similar to endoscopic brow lifting, however, the forehead and the brows are only minimally elevated or repositioned. Instead, the underlying brow and forehead muscles are contoured with a laser to soften the wrinkles, deep lines or creases that have formed. These lines are often associated with a tired and angry look. This is essentially the surgical equivalent of Botox, Xeomin and Dysport. The muscles are surgically weakened to diminish the frown and brow lines just like chemical denervation with Botox, Xeomin and Dysport. Whereas Injectable treatments last for three months, the surgical approach lasts for many years.

Endoscopic Neck Lifting tightens the neck and jaw line. Through small incisions placed behind the ears and under the chin, the underlying fatty tissue in the neck is sculpted through liposuction or 'liposculpture.' During this process the muscles in the neck are also tightened. Through elevating and repositioning the underlying supporting structures, this procedure recreates a more defined neckline and more youthful jaw line.

Endoscopic Midface Lifting accomplishes a lift of the cheek region creating the appearance of a higher and more well-defined cheekbone. In addition the nasolabial fold, the deep fold that runs between the cheek and lip, is softened. Overall, this conveys a more youthful facial appearance for patients concerned with the aging that has happened in these facial regions. Endoscopic midface lifting is not a substitute for a conventional facelift procedure as the neck and temples are not improved by this limited procedure.

CONSIDERING FACELIFT AND NECKLIFT?

a s we age our faces change. This is common knowledge, and no matter what we do we can't avoid it. What you might not know is that the actual shape of your face will also change. The youthful face is heart shaped – wider at the cheeks and midface and gently contoured to a narrower appearance in the lower face. The aged face has a rounder, more inverted heart shape that is instead bottom heavy. People who have an almond shaped face will start to notice their face shifting towards a more oval configuration. An oval face will slowly shift towards a more round shape. The round shaped face will go towards a more square shape. The square shaped face doesn't start to shift to a different shape, but it is the face shape that ages the least gracefully. With a square shaped face even the most minimal loss of fat and wrinkling will be noticeable immediately. Individuals with high cheekbones and an almond shaped face can camouflage laxity of skin and muscle more readily. These people age the most gracefully.

Normally there is a groove that runs from the nose to the corner of the mouth. This line is called the nasolabial fold. This 'fold' is a normal anatomical feature of the face. It is created because of the muscles that form in this area. However, as we age this fold can become more prominent. Many people notice that it starts to extend below the corner of the mouth and begins to form a jowl. Often, this is when people start to look at getting this surgically corrected.

There are two ways of addressing laxity in this midface area. The best way to describe how to change this facial feature is to think of the fold as a hill and valley.

One way to address the problem is to fill in the valley. This is effective. However, this method typically involves fillers and other injectables and is a temporary solution. Most often injectable fillers, fat injections, Live Fill™ or facial implants are used to fill the valley. Live Fill™ is a unique procedure developed at Clevens Face and Body Specialists where Platelet Healing Gel™ is used in combination with the transfer of fat to fill facial lines and folds. Live Fill™ offers the advantages of fat and the unique healing attributes of Platelet Healing Gel™ . These are all outpatient procedures and require very little recovery time. The fillers work well to help preserve or extend a more rested appearance to the face. Often, using the fillers and injectables can postpone the need for facelift surgery. Eventually, the valley will be too deep for the fillers to work and that is when the following option can be looked at.

Rather than filling the valley, one can treat prominence and sagging in this area by reducing or moving the hill. This is essentially a facelift procedure. In this procedure the excess skin would be removed, the lax facial muscles would be tightened, and the area would look more youthful.

This type of facelift procedure is called a rhytidectomy. It is used to treat the neck, cheeks, jowls, and the lateral temporal or eyebrow areas of the face. This procedure creates the most dramatic and long lasting improvement that is possible from facial plastic surgery. It does this because it addresses all the areas of concern at one time. During this procedure, the tissues are repositioned into a more normal, natural, and youthful place. Essentially it helps to turn back the clock approximately ten to twelve years for most people. Studies have shown that many patients feel that they look at least ten years younger after their facelift.

Another issue that comes with the aging process is a loss of moisture from the skin. This leads to the fat redistributing itself. When that happens, both the skin and the muscles become more lax. Facelift surgery can address many of these areas.

Liposuction is often used in conjunction with a facelift surgery to remove excess fatty tissue, including tissue that has repositioned itself. In some cases, fat can herniate down into the jowl area and accentuate fullness where fullness isn't wanted. This is when liposuction can be used to help. It only requires a small incision on the inside of the mouth to remove the excess fatty tissue in this area.

In the youthful neck, the left and right platysma muscles are fused in the midline, creating a sturdy supporting hammock that endows us with a strong, angular chin and neck contour. As we age, the left and right platysma muscles separate in the midline and fall to the side and then sag forward. This laxity of the neck and platysma muscles creates a deep banding and cording appearance in the neck. During facelift surgery, these muscles are placed back into their normal position. This lifting and tightening of the muscles actually re-establishes the neck anatomy that we had in our youth, recreating the strong and sharp neckline of our formative years.

By repositioning these muscles we are able to obtain a more natural appearance. We feel it is important to reposition the muscles and if possible to avoid cutting or altering their position. When the muscles are cut or altered this can create a more artificial appearance and it also requires a longer healing process.

Once the excess fat has been removed and the muscles have been put back into position, there is one last step. During facelift surgery the excess skin is also removed. The sutures are strategically placed to camouflage them.

Newly developed lasers have greatly accelerated the healing associated with facelifts. One of these is the high energy super pulsed laser. Using this tool has helped to reduce the swelling and bruising that is associated with facelift surgery by approximately 60 percent. When using lasers, most individuals are able to return to work and social activities within seven days of the procedure. With a more traditional, conventional facelift there is a two week minimum recovery time.

NEWLY DEVELOPED **LASERS** HAVE GREATLY **ACCELERATED** THE **HEALING** ASSOCIATED WITH FACELIFTS. **ONE OF THESE IS THE HIGH ENERGY SUPER PULSED LASER.**

HOW LONG DOES A
FACELIFT LAST?

n theory, a facelift will last forever because the excess skin has been surgically removed. However, the reality is that we continue to age. One way to think about this process is to think of time as a conveyor belt.

If the surgery takes place at age 50, the individual getting the surgery will look ten years younger. So, although they are chronologically 50, they appear to be 40. But that conveyor belt of time keeps moving forward. If you look at that same individual ten years later, he or she will now be chronologically at the age of 60, but will still look ten years younger, which at this point would be 50. It is for this reason that many people continue to have cosmetic surgeries. However, this is certainly not necessary.

TO HAVE A VERY NATURAL APPEARANCE.

AND THIS ALLOWS PEOPLE TO MAINTAIN THEIR RESULTS AS MUCH AS POSSIBLE.

It should be pointed out that every facelift patient can continue to get improvements by having a tuck-up procedure one year (or more) after the initial surgery is done. This is not a requirement and often people are so pleased with their appearance that they never consider the tuck-up. We think it is important to have a very natural appearance. We work to create a good foundation for surgery and this allows people to maintain their results as much as possible.

SURGICAL TECHNIQUE

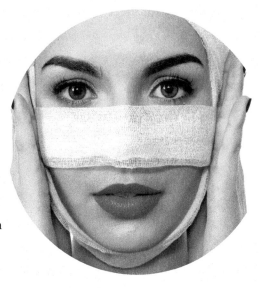

s we have discussed, facial aging is a function of three anatomical processes. There are changes in the skin, muscle and fat. As we age, the skin loses its elasticity and becomes wrinkled. The muscle becomes weak and sags and creates bands and cords in the neck, face and nasolabial fold regions. Fat droops and becomes deposited in unfavorable areas such as the jowl and underneath the chin.

For a facelift to be successful, the anatomical changes of aging must be reversed. A modern facelift does not just tighten the skin. This gives a windblown and unnatural appearance. Instead, the most advanced techniques refinish the skin, reposition and contour unfavorable fat deposits, and tighten the muscles. This creates a natural appearing and long lasting, youthful facelift.

For a female patient, the incisions made are hidden within the skin creases that naturally surround the ear. This means there is no incision in front of the ear, which can be a telltale sign of facelift surgery. The incision will extend from behind the ear back into the hairline. In the frontal temporal area the incision also extends into the hairline. The incisions are closed with dissolvable sutures in multilayers and the hair is not shaved. Small clips are often used in order to allow the patient to shower following surgery. It is also common to have a small incision perhaps two thirds of an inch in length through the natural chin crease below the chin. This helps to obtain additional support and contouring in the neck.

The key to successful facelift surgery is to recreate a natural youthful appearance with techniques that make patients look better and more refreshed, but not different. Incisions should be hidden in places where they are not noticeable.

RECOVERY

ollowing the surgery, a turban-like dressing is used for the first two days and cold compresses are placed over the neck area. The next morning the dressing is removed and cold compresses are applied to the face and neck. This process should continue for at least the next few days. Hydrogen peroxide soaked Q-tips® are used to clean over incision lines. This helps to accelerate wound healing and also to prevent scabs and crusts from forming.

Individuals will need to sleep with their head elevated for two weeks after the procedure. It is also vital to avoid any heavy lifting or straining for the first two to three weeks following surgery. One should also minimize movement of the head and neck for at least one week following surgery to avoid stretching the newly positioned tissues.

It will take a while for you to be able to resume normal activities. Driving, exercise, and other activities that can cause a strain on your muscles need to be avoided for at least one week and potentially longer, depending on your personal healing process. After about one week's time you can start using makeup on your face. But, again, this will depend on your personal healing process. Meticulous technique and attention to detail by the surgeon should allow patients to resume many of their normal activities in ten to fourteen days. You should return to work and play with your friends telling you that you look rested and that perhaps you were on vacation.

CONSIDERING
COSMETIC LASER SKIN RESURFACING?

asers, once thought to be something seen only in science fiction movies, have moved to the forefront of medicine. Cosmetic Laser Skin Resurfacing is a constantly evolving technique that has been around for almost twenty years. In Cosmetic Laser Skin Resurfacing, a laser light is used to virtually 'erase' wrinkles. The laser works in one of two ways depending upon the device and technique chosen. In ablative laser skin resurfacing, the laser removes the most superficial layers of the skin. As it does this it will also be removing many of the skin's imperfections and blemishes. In non-ablative laser skin resurfacing, the laser energy leaves the surface of the skin intact as it passes through to the deeper layers of the skin where it stimulates a new layer of skin to form. Both the ablative and non-ablative techniques stimulate collagen and elastic fiber production in the deeper layers of the skin, which causes your body to begin creating new, fresh looking skin.

The laser resurfacing procedure can be done to one specific region of the face, for example, around the eyes or around the mouth, or it can be done to the full face. Although new, the procedure has been used on tens of thousands of patients all over the world and has proven to be a safe and effective method of removing wrinkles and other signs of aging.

We offer numerous state-of-the-art lasers for cosmetic skin resurfacing at the Clevens Face and Body Specialists. Some lasers emit an intense beam of light that vaporizes tissue instantaneously and with great precision. Other lasers gently pass energy into the deeper layers of the skin, creating a remodeling effect over time. By selecting the proper laser for an individual's skin type and personal concerns, we are able to erase unwanted blemishes, wrinkles, lines, and scarring from your face.

With the ideal laser in hand, we gently remove imperfections in the skin, layer by layer, revealing deeper healthier skin. Since the laser seals blood vessels, lymphatics, and nerve endings, there is very little pain associated with the procedure. Recovery time is very short and there is remarkably little post-operative pain or discomfort. The choice of which laser is appropriate in your individual case is based upon the thorough assessment of your age, skin type, extent of sun damage, and the degree of lines and wrinkle formation that you want to have removed. During a consultation we will go over all of the details for your procedure and how this exciting new modality works.

There are many different types of cosmetic lasers being used. Some of these work well on removing wrinkles, while others work better on scarring. At the Clevens Face and Body Specialists we use lasers that work well on wrinkles, sun damaged skin, acne scarring, removing brown spots, spider veins, rosacea, broken blood vessels, tattoos and even stretch marks.

Of course, there are other methods of skin resurfacing that you can use that don't involve a laser. There are options like microdermabrasion, radiofrequency treatment, blue light, dermabrasion and chemical peels that will create a more youthful look. With each of these techniques, the outer layers of wrinkled and damaged skin are treated to achieve a more refreshed appearance. Similarly, chemical peel techniques also improve facial appearance through the application of special chemical solutions to the top layers of your skin, revealing a more youthful and smooth skin surface. Regardless of the method employed, the goal of all skin resurfacing methods is to minimize the appearance of fine lines and wrinkles. With laser resurfacing there is less bleeding, bruising, and post-operative discomfort than with some of the other resurfacing techniques.

RESURFACING:
COMMONLY ASKED QUESTIONS

What does the laser do?

The laser is a beam of light that vaporizes the outer layers of damaged skin. The laser works at precisely controlled levels of penetration. The old skin layers are erased/removed by the laser and this allows for the fresh, new skin underneath to shine through. After healing, the skin on the face appears tighter, smoother, and younger looking.

What are the most common uses for laser skin resurfacing?

Examples of the most common skin issues that are treated with laser skin resurfacing are as follows: removal of facial wrinkles, removal of deep lines around the mouth and eyes, treatment of facial scars, treatment of scarring related to acne, treatment of areas of uneven skin pigmentation, removal of tattoos, and treatment of precancerous skin conditions.

Who are the best candidates for laser skin resurfacing?

Although this modality is available for men and women of all ages and skin types, not everyone is ideal for this procedure. Traditionally, the ideal patient for skin resurfacing has fair, healthy, non-oily skin. But, newer laser techniques now allow us to safely and effectively treat even patients with darker skin tones such as olive, brown, or black skin. As always, enhancement of your skin is the goal. Perfection and a complete removal of all facial skin flaws may not be realistic. The reality is that lines or creases that are a result of the facial skin muscles, "smiling, squinting, talking, blinking," are eventually going to come back.

Does it hurt? Is anesthesia necessary?

There is a certain amount of discomfort that is experienced with laser resurfacing. When a full face procedure is done, twilight or mild sedation is often used. With a regional resurfacing, around the mouth or eyes, often a local anesthetic will be used. During the first few hours and days after the procedure, there is usually mild burning and discomfort, which feels much like a sunburn. Oral painkillers and ice packs help control the discomfort.

How long does the procedure take?

The procedure is relatively quick. However, the amount of time that it will take is going to be directly connected to the amount of damaged skin that requires removal and the size of the area being treated. In general, a regional resurfacing will only take about fifteen minutes, while a treatment of the full face can take about one hour.

How long does it take to heal?

This really depends upon the type of laser selected and whether we have decided to perform ablative or non-ablative resurfacing. During your healing process, new collagen and elastic fibers are formed. The laser requires the skin to rebuild itself from the bottom up.

How long does laser resurfacing last?

According to most of the studies that have been done on laser skin resurfacing, the treatments can permanently improve the color, texture, and lines of the face. It is believed that these long- term changes happen because the laser encourages the production of collagen and elastic fibers in the deeper layers of the skin. This creates a more vibrant and youthful appearance for many years to come.

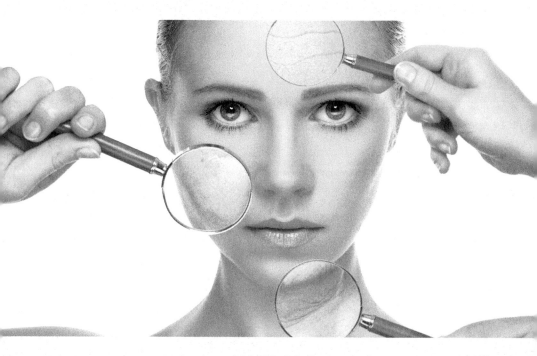

CONSIDERING RHINOPLASTY OR NASAL CONTOURING?

asal surgery, also referred to as rhinoplasty, is one of the most frequently performed facial plastic surgical procedures. It is done not only for appearance but also to improve breathing. The nose has multiple growth centers and doesn't mature until we reach puberty.

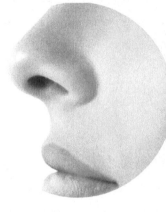

Childhood trauma can damage these growth centers, with the end result being a crooked nose, either internally, externally, or both. Some people seek out nasal surgery for a more recent injury. Others seek nasal surgery to change an unwanted ethnic or family trait that was obtained through inherited genes. Fortunately, facial plastic surgery can help to correct any of these issues.

WHAT WILL YOU LOOK LIKE?

he nose is an individual characteristic. For many, the most attractive nose is one that is natural and proportional for the face. The size and shape of the nose that looks right for the attractive model in a magazine may not look right on your face. It may not be the right proportion for your face. It is important that the nose be both symmetrical and proportional.

The distance between the tip of the nose and the base should ideally equal the distance from the base to the upper lip. The most ideal angle between the nose and the upper lip, also called the nasolabial angle, should be between 95 to 110 degrees. The base of the nose should fall within the plane of two lines drawn perpendicular from the inner aspect of each eye. The above is what is considered the ideal proportion for the nose. This is going to be individual for each person. In order to know exactly what you would look like once your nose has been improved, we can show you using state of the art computer programs that we use. The above is what is considered the ideal proportion for the nose. This is going to be individual for each person. In order to know exactly what you would look like once your nose has been improved, we can show you using state of the art computer programs that we use.

ANATOMY

he nose consists of bone, cartilage, and skin. The aesthetic that is possible on your face is limited to a large extent by the strength, tone, and shape of these tissues. Just as an artist is limited by the quality of the materials that are available, so too is the facial surgeon limited by the patient's tissues and underlying structure.

Internally, you can think of your nose as an A-frame house. There is a middle partition that divides the nose, or house, into two equal parts. This middle partition is called the septum. Unfortunately, it is common for this middle partition to be asymmetrical.

If the septum is deviated, widened, or thickened, it can result in airway obstruction. This is what people are referring to when they talk about having a deviated septum.

The function of the nose is to warm the air, increase humidification of air, and filter out impurities. Part of this is done by the lining of the nose, which is not straight. There are actually three projections on each side of the nose called turbinates. These projections provide additional surface area for the nose to perform its functions. These turbinates can become abnormally enlarged due to trauma or inhalation allergies. If they enlarge too much they can obstruct the airflow and the drainage passages that lead to the sinuses.

The result of these blockages can lead to sinus headaches or infections. Many times the turbinates will swell at night when one is reclined. Mouth breathing, snoring, sore throats in the morning, chronic nasal congestion, posterior nasal drainage, and nose bleeds can all be signs of nasal deformity. These deformities can be decreased or eliminated with nasal surgery.

IN ORDER TO KNOW EXACTLY **WHAT YOU WOULD LOOK LIKE** ONCE YOUR NOSE HAS BEEN IMPROVED, **WE CAN SHOW YOU USING STATE OF THE ART COMPUTER PROGRAMS THAT WE USE.**

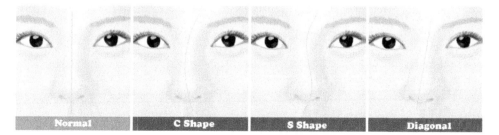

Normal   C Shape   S Shape   Diagonal

HOW SURGERY IS PERFORMED

t is most common for surgical incisions to be made inside of the nose; although, on occasion, an incision will need to be made at the base of the nose or at the base of the nostrils. However, these incisions are usually undetectable when fully healed.

The mucosal lining that exists over the septum is lifted off the nasal structure using special instruments. With this lining out of the way, it is easier to identify the deformity and irregularity of bones and cartilage. Through small incisions made inside the nose, the external abnormalities can be contoured. Small instruments are used to make incisions in the bones and cartilage to reshape enlarged or twisted structures. The bones and cartilage are then repositioned to improve the nasal airway.

In some cases the nose is packed, although this can be avoided in most instances with careful attention to detail and special suturing techniques inside the nose. Packing can cause some discomfort after the procedure as it creates more pressure in the surgical site. It also requires the packing to be removed, which is an uncomfortable process. Luckily the packing process can often be avoided if dissolvable sutures are used to reposition tissues. This technique may be more difficult than packing the nose, but it is much more accurate and it avoids the problems associated with pain and pressure from the packing. A nasal dressing consisting of a custom-conforming plastic splint is left in place for approximately one week to help mold the bones and cartilage into the desired shape.

RECOVERY

t is important to minimize the amount of swelling and bruising following surgery. It is for this reason that a dressing, which covers the eyes and nose, is commonly applied for the first twenty- four hours following surgery. After the dressing is removed, ice compresses are applied and should be continued for at least the next two days.

At the end of one week, the last of the dressing is typically removed. This is done by applying a special liquid to the dressing, which loosens the tape and allows the bandage to be removed without any discomfort for the patient. The nose will still be swollen, but it will be possible to see the basic changes that have been made to the nose. The changes will be more noticeable and significant as the nose fully heals over the next twelve months. Ninety percent of individuals can see a positive change at one week following surgery. However, approximately ten percent of individual's experience swelling and bruising that can last for a number of weeks.

It actually takes up to one full year for the nose to completely heal, but around three to four months after the surgery the changes will be the most obvious. Up through the four- month mark the nasal structure will be fragile as it mends and heals. It is for this reason that all contact sports, diving, and other potentially dangerous activities should be avoided. After all the effort related to your nasal surgery, you certainly do not want to undo the good work that has been done.It is important to avoid wearing glasses of any kind for the first four to six weeks after surgery. The constant gentle pressure of glasses can result in slight movement or repositioning of the nasal bones. Individuals who need to wear glasses in order to see will be required to wear a protective splint. This will help to avoid putting pressure on the healing nasal bones.

Following nasal surgery, it is ideal to sleep with the head elevated for at least two weeks. Sleeping with the head higher than the heart helps to markedly decrease the amount of swelling and bruising. Lifting more than five to ten pounds for the first two weeks is also prohibited following surgery.

During this time frame it is also important to avoid any activities that cause the heart rate to accelerate. Increased blood pressure could result in more swelling and this increases the possibility of developing a nosebleed. Blowing the nose for the first two weeks following rhinoplasty surgery should also be avoided. If you must sneeze, do it with an open mouth in order to minimize the irritation to the healing nasal tissues.

Following surgery, ice compresses are used for the first two to three days. Ice packs should not be used as they are too heavy and do not get into the creases of the face. A better option is to use washcloths that have been soaked in ice water. These can then be folded into an inverted 'V' configuration and fit right into the area that needs the ice pack. They can be easily draped over the nose and contour over these areas. Ideally the ice packs should be changed every ten minutes for maximum results.

A drip pad, or mustache dressing, is also commonly applied after surgery. This is simply a gauze square that serves to collect any drainage from the nose. It is not uncommon to have to change this several times during the first few hours after surgery. After several days a drip pad may not be necessary. However, if there is continual drainage, it is better to use the drip pad, rather than dab the nose with a facial tissue. Individuals should not fly for at least several days following their nasal surgery. During a flight, there are marked changes in the air pressure of the airplane and this change in pressure can cause a nosebleed. It can also affect the face mask that is used to regulate the pressure on the face. It is better to avoid this potentially problematic situation. It is normal to have some swelling and congestion following nasal surgery. This usually persists for several weeks. Most people experience improvement in their breathing after the first few days following the surgery. Breathing should continue to improve as the nose fully heals. Keep in mind that the final result of the nasal surgery, both internally and externally, is not achieved until up to one year following the procedure. Often people will use various types of oral antihistamines and nasal sprays, which serve to accelerate the healing process and dissipate any problems with nasal congestion.

ADDITIONAL PROCEDURES

IT ACTUALLY TAKES **UP TO ONE FULL YEAR** FOR THE **NOSE TO COMPLETELY HEAL**, BUT AROUND **THREE TO FOUR MONTHS AFTER THE SURGERY** THE **CHANGES WILL BE THE MOST OBVIOUS.**

ften individuals want additional facial surgical procedures performed at the same time as nasal surgery. This combination of surgeries allows less time away from work and social activities because the recovery of each operation is done simultaneously. There is also some reduction in cost because you avoid various duplicate fees such as operating room facility fees, lab test fees, anesthesia, supply fees, and the cost of medications.

Most facial plastic surgical procedures can be performed in conjunction with rhinoplasty surgery; however, dermabrasion and chemical face peeling cannot. With skin resurfacing procedures, patients are often required to shower in order to avoid the formation of scabs and crusting on recently peeled tissues. With nasal surgery, a dressing is applied to mold and shape the nasal tissues for the first week after surgery. Frequent showering could result in displacement of the nasal dressing and must be avoided. However, blepharoplasty surgery, facelifts, cheek and chin implants, and hair transplant surgery can all be performed in conjunction with nasal surgery.

CONSIDERING LASER LIPOSUCTION?

he Smartlipo TriPlex laser is the latest generation of our laser liposuction workstations. The Clevens Face and Body Specialists is proud to offer this new solid state platform Nd:YAG laser capable of emitting laser energy in three wavelengths: 1064 nm, 1320 nm and 1440 nm. These versatile wavelengths can be used independently or can be uniquely blended using our MultiPlex™ technology. This brings our patients the latest and greatest in laser liposuction and skin tightening capabilities.

he ability to customize the sequential firing of wavelengths in combination achieves optimal results by targeting both the fat and water in fatty tissue for more efficient elimination of the fatty tissue while coagulating the skin to optimize tightening effects. This unique laser also targets blood vessels to minimize bruising and speed recovery. This one device enables us to gently dissolve fat without traumatic conventional liposuction while tightening skin and gently sealing blood vessels.

Based on the setting and the motion of the handpiece, the precise laser power is metered and delivered. For added safety, the hand piece senses the motion of the surgeon and either adds or diminishes the power of the laser to keep up with the tempo of the surgeon. This adds reliability enhancing the outcome for our patients.

The Smartlipo TriPlex/Cellulaze workstation offers users a light-based solution not only for unwanted fat but also for cellulite. The Cellulaze workstation is configured with the 1440-nm wavelength and includes a Cellulaze delivery system. At the present time, this is the only proven and FDA approved method of permanent cellulite reduction available in the United States. This unique system offers our patients dramatic and permanent cellulite reduction in a single treatment that can be performed with the safety of local anesthesia in the office setting.

Tissue shrinkage and skin tightening with SmartLipo and Cellulaze is generally between 17-22%. What this means for you, the patient, is that we are able to insert a slender laser beneath your skin and selectively target the collagen fibers to achieve a non-surgical and minimally invasive 20% shrink wrap of the skin in the treated region. In many cases, this avoids the need to cut away excess skin as is often done, for example, in a facelift procedure. So, some patients are eligible for laser dissolution of fat combined with skin tightening instead of a facelift. In the right patient, recovery times can be reduced from 2 weeks to just a few days.

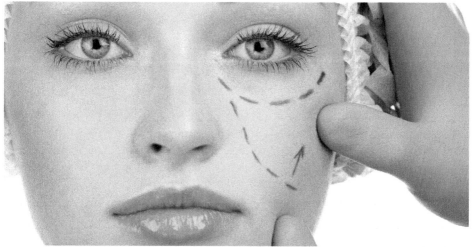

CONSIDERING
THE WEEKEND
STEM CELL FACELIFT™?

magine harnessing the power of stem cell therapy to improve your appearance. Through the science of Platelet Healing Gel™, Dr. Clevens activates your own stem cells to grow new, younger looking skin.

STEM CELL TECHNOLOGY IS UNIQUELY BLENDED WITH HYALURONIC ACID THERAPY AND THE MOST ADVANCED NON-ABLATIVE FRACTIONAL LASER SKIN RESURFACING

The Clevens Face and Body Specialists proudly pioneered the use of Platelet Rich Plasma in facial plastic surgery. Since 2001, Dr. Clevens has improved aesthetic results for over 10,000 patients with autologous unipotent stem cell technology.

The Weekend Stem Cell Facelift™ is a revolutionary facial rejuvenation system that does not involve surgery. At the Clevens Face and Body Specialists, stem cell technology is uniquely blended with hyaluronic acid therapy and the most advanced non-ablative fractional laser skin resurfacing to create a natural result. In the majority of cases, patients exhibit a renewed luminance of their skin, a youthful enhancement in facial contour and a restoration of age-related volume loss.

Performed under comfortable local anesthesia in our office of trusted professionals, The Weekend Stem Cell Facelift™ allows most patients to return to work and their busy lifestyles within one to two days. Before you know it, you'll be looking fresher and years younger. Unleash a more youthful and vibrant "you" with the help of this groundbreaking treatment.

The Weekend Stem Cell Facelift™ is often combined with other procedures to enhance your result. Patients find that Stem Cell Lifting may be joined with laser technologies or filler techniques to create a more youthful appearance with very little downtime. The art of plastic surgery involves combining state of the art techniques in a unique fashion to achieve natural results with less downtime. Recognizing that patients lead busy lives, it is this sort of progressive and creative blending of technologies that leads to better results with less recovery time.

CONSIDERING
LIP ENHANCEMENT?

t is no coincidence that many of today's celebrities have full, sexy lips. Even the ones with naturally thin lips often have lip augmentation in order to achieve the perfect pout. Since ancient times, women have used cosmetics to enhance the appearance of their lips. Full lips have always been a sign of youth and beauty. However, as we age, lips tend to get thinner due to diminishing levels of collagen in the skin. Lips may also wrinkle making you look and feel older than you really appear. Fortunately, lip augmentation is available to give you fuller, younger, sensual looking lips and to help improve your self confidence.

Lip augmentation is becoming increasingly popular because of its speedy recovery time and quick results. Candidates for lip augmentation include: thin lips, wrinkled lips due to aging or smoking, asymmetrical lips or those in need of lip reconstruction.

The lips are the first thing that most people notice about women. One of the most popular aesthetic procedures is lip enhancement. The cosmetic industry recognizes that women spend billions of dollars on their lips, from lipstick to aesthetic injectables. Most augment their lips with injectable fillers, which are repeated about once a year or even more often. Although lip augmentation with fillers is an ideal procedure for adding volume to thin lips, it is not permanent. For a more permanent solution there are several options. These options include fat injections, direct lip lift, sub-nasal lip lift and corner lip lift.

An excellent technique for lip augmentation is fat injections. It offers the only natural method for potential permanent results. Fat is aspirated from another part of the body, such as the abdomen, and then injected into the lips. Since fat cells are living tissue, the body will recognize them and new capillaries will attach to the cells to keep them permanently alive. Since the fat cells are from the patient's own body, they are not recognized as foreign and will not cause an allergic reaction. The fat transfer technique may require two to three treatments to achieve a permanent result as the body absorbs much of the injected fat.

Direct Lip Lift is another option. A direct lip lift surgery removes tissue directly from above the upper lip line border. The end result is a slightly raised effect.

A **Subnasal Lip Lift** is arguably the most popular method of lip lift surgery. This procedure is performed by removing a bit of skin tissue from underneath the nose. When the incision is closed, the removed tissue creates a slight lift in the upper lip.

Depending on the natural shape of their lips, patients may want to combine lip lift surgery with a corner lip lift. Since the fat injections, direct lip lift and the subnasal lip lift techniques don't specifically lift the corners of the mouth, the corner lip lift can help create a more uniform lip line post procedure. The corner lip lift uses tiny incisions above the outer corners of the mouth to subtly raise and even the overall mouth contour. This can prevent lip lift patients from winding up with a slightly downturned lip line. Lip augmentation can be an excellent compliment to many plastic surgical procedures. It can be performed in conjunction with a facelift, forehead/brow lift, laser resurfacing, rhinoplasty, and with facial implants.

CONSIDERING
DERMABRASION?

ermabrasion is a controlled surgical scraping of the skin's top layers. This is done to help soften sharp edges and to correct any irregularities. In our practice, dermabrasion is currently most often used to improve scars after prior reconstructive procedures such as after Mohs surgery for skin cancer or after an injury. The goal of dermabrasion is to create a smoother and more youthful appearance to the skin. This process is often used to correct scarring or smooth out wrinkles. It can also be used to remove pre-cancerous growths, moles and skin irregularities.

The dermabrasion procedure can be done on any area of the body, but is most often performed on the face. It can be done as a stand-alone treatment or in conjunction with other procedures for facial correction.

Most often dermabrasion is done as an outpatient procedure in a surgical facility. Occasionally, if extensive work is being done, it might require a stay in the hospital, but this is a rare occurrence.

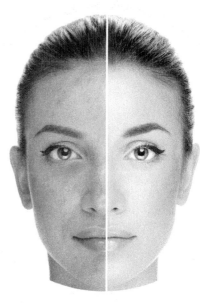

The dermabrasion procedure is typically performed while you are under a local anesthetic. This numbs the area that will be worked on and makes you drowsy, but you are awake for the procedure. There is minimal discomfort, especially when a local anesthetic is used. If, after the local anesthesia is administered and there is still some discomfort, we can also use a numbing spray on the skin.

Overall the process is very quick. The duration can last anywhere from a few minutes to an hour. This will mainly depend on the amount of area that needs to be covered. Sometimes we will recommend that the process be done in stages. This is typically when there is deep scarring or a large area that we need to work on.

During the procedure we are literally scraping away the top layers of skin. This is done with a small burr that has diamond particles on it. The instrument scrapes the layers of skin until we get to a point where the scar or the wrinkle is less noticeable.

There can be some redness and swelling that develops after a treatment. This typically subsides after a few days. You might be given an ointment to place on the treated area for several weeks following the procedure. This is used to help the healing process and to keep the skin clean. You will need to avoid putting anything on the treated area for at least a week.

DERMABRASION
CLOSE-UP

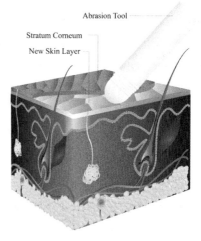

Abrasion Tool

Stratum Corneum

New Skin Layer

CONSIDERING
CHEMICAL PEEL?

there are several different forms of chemical peel that can be used to treat minor wrinkles and discoloration on the face. A chemical peel is the process of using chemical agents to burn the top layers of skin off of the face and potentially other areas of the body.

The peel will leave the skin looking smoother and younger because it takes off the damaged top layers of the skin. This system is one of the easiest ways to improve the appearance of the skin.

The following are skin issues that can be improved with using the chemical peel:

Acne scars

Acne

Fine lines and fine wrinkles

Freckles

Irregular pigmentation

Rough skin

Scars

Sun damage

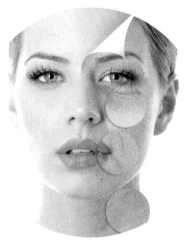

The main chemicals that are used in a chemical peel are phenol, trichloroacetic acid, and alphahydroxy acid. Each of these works at a different strength, and each can be adjusted and mixed with other agents, depending on what your specific needs are. We will work with you to determine the exact mix that you need to make changes to your skin.

There are several different strengths of chemical peel that can be used and each one has its own unique purposes.

Light Chemical Peel

The mildest form of a chemical peel is called a light chemical peel. This version is for the removal of the outer layer of skin and the process will provide a light exfoliation. Most often the light chemical peel is a mixture of alphahydroxy acid and beta hydroxy acid. As this is a mild chemical peel, the treatment can be repeated weekly for up to six weeks in order to get the results that you want. The light chemical peel is not going to remove deep wrinkles, dark spotting, or scarring.

The process is done as an outpatient procedure and is most often done without the need of anesthetic. To begin, your face will be cleaned and then the chemical solution will be brushed onto your skin. There can be a mild stinging sensation while the chemical goes to work. The chemical peel is then washed off.

Medium Depth Chemical Peel

The next strength of chemical peel is the medium chemical peel. This solution is used to deal with acne scars, deeper wrinkling, and uneven skin color. This stronger chemical peel will remove the skin cells that are on the outer layer and the upper part of the middle layer of skin. Most often the acids used for the medium chemical peel are trichloroacetic acid and glycolic acid.

The process is done as an outpatient procedure and is most often carried out with a local anesthetic. After your face is cleaned, the chemical solution will be brushed on to your face for only a few minutes. It is likely that you will feel stinging or burning while the chemical is on your skin. The chemicals are then neutralized with a saline compress.

After a medium peel, your skin will likely turn red and will be highly sensitive. It can take up to six weeks for your skin to stop being red and uncomfortable. The process can be repeated every six months to one year in order for your skin to have that youthful glow.

Deep Chemical Peel

The strongest chemical peel that you can get is called a deep chemical peel. This chemical peel can be used to treat the deepest damage to your facial skin. It can remove sun damage, scarring, discoloration, and even pre-cancerous growth. The chemical used for this chemical peel is phenol.

This process is typically done as an outpatient procedure, but a local anesthetic and a sedative is used to help with discomfort. Unlike the other chemical peels, the deep chemical peel will require a pre-treatment process of up to eight weeks. This will help your skin get ready for the treatment and speed up the healing process.

A medical aesthetician working with your physician will oversee your skin care in preparation for chemical peel. Most often the pretreatment is going to include the use of Retin-A, which is a prescription form of Vitamin A or any one of a variety of other skin care regimens. Each doctor and aesthetician has his or her own preferred method of preparing the skin for chemical peel. Some doctors have even developed their own skin care lines to provide their patients with the best in aesthetic care. This treatment thins out the surface layer of skin and allows the chemical to get deeper and more evenly into the skins levels. After the pretreatment is completed, you will come into the office for the chemical peel. During your peel, a special chemical solution is brushed onto the skin. The solution that is used depends upon the depth and the type of chemical peel that is most appropriate for you. As noted above, some peels are light (glycolic acids, 10-20% tricholoracetic acid [TCA]), medium (25-45% trichloroacetic [TCA]) or deep (phenol or Baker's solution) The timing that is required will depend on what your skin issues are and what type of peel is selected. The chemical can be left for anywhere between 10 minutes and one hour. When the process is completed, some peels are neutralized with water and others are just left to be as is.

After neutralization or completion of the peel, your skin will be coated with petroleum jelly. It must remain on your skin for one to two days in order to help the skin stay moisturized during the healing process. During the first few days the skin will start peel. Crusting and scabbing should be avoided as this can lead to scarring or unwanted blotchiness, lightening or darkening of the skin (hyperpigmentation or hypopigmentation). There will be redness, peeling, and burning for several days after a deep chemical peel procedure. Most often, patients deal with this discomfort with painkillers. The swelling will subside within two weeks, but the skin could stay red for up to three months. Although the healing process takes several months, one deep chemical peel treatment can last for up to ten years.

CONSIDERING
ANTI-AGING PHYSICIAN GRADE SKIN CARE?

emerging from 15 years of clinical research and experience, Dr. Ross Clevens has created his own premiere skin care product line. Inspired by excellence in innovation, this unique line stimulates cellular rejuvenation and builds collagen to create smooth and radiant skin. This new skin care line is exclusive to Clevens Face and Body Specialists and is specially formulated through the beauty of science to deliver results.

We are committed to offering only the best in skin care solutions to help maintain your surgical investment. Many individuals who are not our surgical patients take advantage of these same products to improve the appearance of their skin. Other doctors have also created their own unique skin care lines. Many forms of skin care feel good; but physician grade skin care is often prescription strength and able to deliver real results.

In our practice, licensed medical aestheticians will gladly customize your experience with an effective combination of products to meet your individual needs. In our experience, a professionally supervised skin care regimen is highly effective and often more economical than products you might buy online or in a department store.

The Clevens Skin Care Line features pure botanicals and rich antioxidants that diminish the appearance of fine lines. A combination of soap-free cleansers, ultra-pure glycolic acid, detoxifying mint, Vitamins A, C, E, CoQ-10, Green Tea and Tea Tree Oil ensures a flawlessly beautiful complexion.

CONSIDERING RADIOFREQUENCY (RF) SKIN TIGHTENING AND REJUVENATION?

Certain skin treatment devices use electrical pulses in the radiofrequency range to target specific areas of the skin and fatty tissues beneath the skin. The RF pulses penetrate the skin and stimulate the tissues creating tightening and smoothing. It is proven that as RF energy passes into the deeper layers of the skin, dermal heating results and this has an immediate effect on collagen structure resulting in skin tightening. Over the longer term, this stimulates the skin to create renewed collagen in a process known as neocollagenesis resulting in improved skin texture and decrease in wrinkles. Early RF devices were painful, but current generation technology is able to focus the energy using three dimensional (3D) precision in a nearly painless manner.

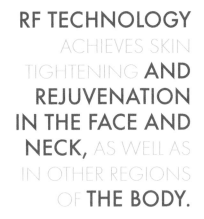

RF TECHNOLOGY ACHIEVES SKIN TIGHTENING **AND REJUVENATION IN THE FACE AND NECK,** AS WELL AS IN OTHER REGIONS OF **THE BODY.**

3D Technology employs a multi-source, phase-controlled radio frequency energy that is state-of-the-art, safe and effective. The latest generation in the evolution of RF-based professional skin treatment devices achieves improved tightening and resurfacing with no significant downtime. The selective use of multiple RF sources and sophisticated software controls the phase of the energy so the treatment is painless and safe.

3D RF treatments are typically performed as a series of between four and six treatments at intervals every week or two. Sessions are performed in the office and no anesthesia or sedation is necessary as the treatments are painless. RF technology achieves skin tightening and rejuvenation in the face and neck, as well as in other regions of the body. In the face and neck, three dimensional radio-frequency energy smooths and tightens the lower eyelids and crow's feet, lifts the jowls and contours the chin and neckline. In the body, RF improves cellulite and tightens the arms, tummy and thighs. Current 3D RF technology is a non-surgical minimally invasive technology with no downtime that provides a glimpse into the future world of incision-less and scar-less cosmetic surgery.

CONSIDERING
PERMANENT MAKEUP?

ermanent makeup is a technique involving a medical grade micropigmentation tattoo. It creates a natural look of carefully applied makeup. With permanent makeup you can enjoy the benefits of looking great from the moment you wake up in the morning. It can mimic eyeliner, eyebrow pencil, lip liner, and lipstick. Imagine, with permanent makeup, you can wake up to a new day, look in the mirror and your makeup has already been applied. Whether swimming, exercising, or playing sports, your makeup is always perfect. No more struggling with drawing eyebrows, only to have them smear off or getting a perfect eyeliner, just to wind up with black eyes. Permanent makeup is ideal for on-the-go women who want to look their best. Permanent makeup is nice for women who cannot afford the time nor wish to take the time to apply makeup throughout the day. No more worries of reapplying lipstick all day, just to have it bleed into those fine wrinkles. At the end of the day, your makeup looks as though it had just been freshened. ■

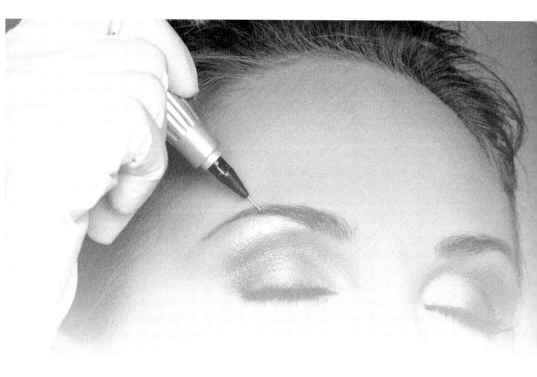

YOUR **NOTES**

_____

_____

_____

_____

_____

_____

_____

_____

_____

_____

_____

_____

_____

_____

_____

_____

_____

_____

_____

YOUR NOTES

EPILOGUE:
A JOURNEY OF A THOUSAND MILES STARTS WITH A SINGLE STEP

n this book we have discussed that your facial plastic surgery experience is a journey, not a destination. It has been your journey to find the right surgeon, to select the right procedure and to enjoy the well-deserved fruits of your procedure. The last thousand miles that have been your cosmetic journey is over. What an accomplishment! You did it! It's over! All your dreams, all your planning, all your efforts have finally come to fruition. But, this does not bring us to the end. 3D Technology employs a multi-source, phase-controlled radio frequency energy that is state-of-the-art, safe and effective. The latest generation in the evolution of RF-based professional skin treatment devices achieves improved tightening and resurfacing with no significant downtime. The selective use of multiple RF sources and sophisticated software controls the phase of the energy so the treatment is painless and safe.

By now you have realized that this final step is not really final at all; instead, you have embarked on a lifestyle process that should never end. Your journey of the next thousand miles begins. The first step to your improved future has been your cosmetic surgery adventure. You are confident with the new you and its lifetime effects, both physically and psychosocially. You have incorporated this healthy skin-smart knowledge into your way of living. This is now second nature. Indeed, you have come a long way.

You started out by not knowing for sure what you even wanted; but through curiosity, investigation, inquiry, and research, you took that first wary step into the world of facial plastic surgery. You began your journey with the one-on-one confidence-building meeting with your patient concierge. This led to your confidential conversation with your facial plastic surgeon during which you shared your most intimate concerns about your appearance.

I n consultation with your facial plastic surgery specialist in The Specialist Advantage, you created your unique aesthetic game plan to secure your aesthetic dreams. You then prepared for your special day by making preparations and plodding through the Reassurance Program, reviewing your personal health history, completing necessary paperwork and finalizing your financial investment.

Then your big day of your Tailor Made Surgery arrived at the ambulatory surgical center. You met with your surgical nurse who was with you throughout the entire operation. You talked with the anesthesiologist and finally with your surgeon to address last minute concerns. You were whisked into surgery and then, seemingly a moment later, were recovered and headed home to convalesce. You were comforted during the next phase, The Nurturing Process, knowing that your healthcare team was always on call for you, night and day.

You transitioned seamlessly from the Nurturing Process to the next phase, the Image Maximizer where you learned about maintaining and enhancing your investment with confidence and strength. The next step in your great odyssey is the Image Expander – only to find that it's not a final step at all but a launch into a lifestyle of health and well-being – the next thousand miles.

As your doctor, as your teacher, and as your friend, I would like to thank you for allowing me to accompany you on your travels through *A Consumer's Guide to Facial Plastic Surgery, Your Facial Surgery Companion*. I wish you all the best in the continuation of your journey forward and hope that we meet again soon.

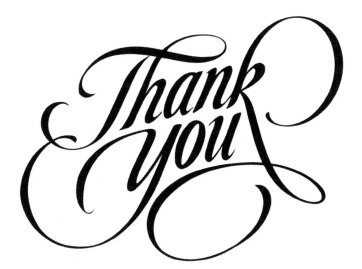

MEDICATIONS TO
AVOID BEFORE AND
AFTER SURGERY

our surgeon may advise you to avoid certain medications around the time of your surgery. In our practice, if you are taking any medication(s) on this list, you are advised to discontinue these starting two weeks prior to surgery. Only Tylenol should be taken for pain unless otherwise specifically instructed. We ask our patients to inform us of all medications they are currently taking. It is important that each medication you take is specifically approved by your doctor.

ASPIRIN MEDICATIONS TO AVOID

4-Way Cold Tabs
5-Aminosalicylic Acid
Acetylsalicylic Acid
Adprin-B products
Alka-Seltzer products
Amigesic
Anacin products
Anexsia w/Codeine
Argesic-SA
Arthra-G
Arthriten products
Arthritis Foundation
    products
Arthritis Pain Formula
Arthritis Strength BC
    Powder
Arthropan
ASA
Asacol
Ascriptin products
Aspergum Azdone
Asprimox products
Axotal
Azulfidine products
B-A-C
Backache Maximum

Strength Relief
Bayer Products
BC Powder
Bismatrol products
Buffered Aspirin
Bufferin products
Buffetts 11
Buffex
Butal/ASA/Caff
Butalbital Compound
Cama Arthritis Pain
    Reliever
Carisoprodol Compound
Cheracol
Choline Magnesium
    Trisalicylate
Choline Salicylate
Cope
Coricidin
Cortisone Medications
Damason-P
Darvon Compound-65
DarvonIA SA
Dipentum
Disalcid
Doan's product

Dolobid
Dristan
Duragesic
Easprin
Ecotrin products Excedrin
    products
Empirin products
Equagesic
Fiorgen PF
Fiorinal products
Gelpirin
Genprin
Gensan
Goody's Extra Strength
    Headache Powders
Halfrin products
Isollyl Improved
Kaodene
Lanorinal
Lortab ASA
Magan Magsal
Magnaprin products
Magnesium Salicylate
    Marthritic
Marnal
Meprobamate

Mesalamine
Methocarbamol
Micrainin
Mobidin
Mobigesic
Momentum
Mono-Gesic
Night-Time Effervescent
    Cold
Norgesic products
Norwich products
Olsalazine
Orphengesic products
Oxycodone
Pabalate products
P-A-C
Pain Reliever Tabs
Panasal
Pentasa

Pepto-Bismol
Percodan products
Phenaphenl Codeine #3
Pink Bismuth
Propoxyphene Compound
    products
Robaxisal
Rowasa
Roxeprin
Saleto products
Salfiex
Salicylate products
Salsalate
Salsitab
Scot-Tussin Original
    5-Action
Sine-off
Sinutab
Sodium Salicylate

Sodol Compound
Soma Compound
St. Joseph Aspirin
Sulfasalazine
Supac
Suprax
Synalgos-DC
Taiwin
Triaminicin
Tricosal
Trilisate
Tussanil DR
Tussirex products
Ursinus-Inlay
Vanquish
Wesprin
Willow Bark products
Zorprin

IBUPROFEN AND NSAID MEDICATIONS TO AVOID

Actron
Acular (opthalmic)
Advil products
Aleve
Anaprox products
Ansaid
Cataflam
Clinoril
Daypro
Diclofenac
Dimetapp Sinus
Dristan Sinus
Etodolac
Feldene
Fenoprofen
Flurbiprofen
Genpril
Haltran
IBU

Ibuprin
Ibuprofen
Indochron E-R
Indocin products
Indomethacin products
Ketoprofen
Ketorolac
lbuprohm
Lodine
Meclofenamate
Meclomen
Mefenamic Acid
Menadol
Midol products
Motrin products
Nabumetone
Nalfon products
Naprelan
Naprosyn products

Naprox X
Naproxen
Nuprin
Ocufen (opthalmic)
Orudis products
Oruvail
Oxaprozin
Piroxicam
Ponstel
Profenal
Relafen
Rhinocaps
Sine-Aid products
Sulindac
Suprofen
Tolectin products
Tolmetin
Toradol
Voltaren

TRICYCLIC ANTIDEPRESSANTS MEDICATIONS TO AVOID

Adapin	Endep	Pertofrane
Amitriptyline	Etrafon products	Protriptyline
Amoxapine	Imipramine	Sinequan
Anafranil	Janimine	Surmontil
Asendin	Limbitrol products	Tofranil
Aventyl	Ludiomil	Triavil
Clomipramine	Maprotiline	Trimipramine
Desipramine	Norpramin	Vivactil
Doxepin	Nortriptyline	
Elavil	Pamelor	

OTHER MEDICATIONS TO AVOID

4-Way w/ Codeine	Enoxaparin injection	Pyrroxate
A.C.A.	Flagyl	Ru-Tuss
A-A Compound	Fragmin injection	Salatin
Accutrim	Furadantin	Sinex
Actifed	Garlic	Sofarin
Anexsia	Heparin	Soltice
Anisindione	Hydrocortisone	Sparine
Anturane	Isollyl	Stelazine
Arthritis Bufferin	Lovenox injection	Sulfinpyrazone
BC Tablets	Macrodantin	Tenuate
Childrens Advil	Mellaril	Tenuate Dospan
Clinoril C	Miradon	Thorazine
Contac	Opasal	Ticlid
Coumadin	Pan-PAC	Ticlopidine
Dalteparin injection	Pentoxyfylline	Trental
Dicumerol	Persantine	Ursinus
Dipyridamole	Phenyipropanolamine	Vibramycin
Doxycycline	Prednisone	Vitamin E
Emagrin	Protamine	Warfarin

HERBAL MEDICATIONS TO AVOID

Arnica	Ginseng	Vitamin A
Bromelain	Kava Kava	Vitamin E
Fish oil	Melatonin	
Ginkgo Biloba	St. Johns Wort	

A FINAL WORD
ON SMOKING

discuss with each patient the fact that the use of tobacco adversely affects all aspects of an individual's health and well-being and that smoking is problematic in facial plastic surgery, as well. I inform the patient that it impairs wound healing, causing significant adverse outcomes, and increases the complication rate in elective facial plastic surgery and in facial cosmetic surgery.

I recommend that the patient stop smoking for a minimum of two weeks, and preferably four weeks, prior to the surgical procedure and to remain tobacco-free for a minimum of two weeks, and preferably four weeks, after the surgical procedure, highlighting that patients who are not willing to stop smoking around the time of surgery have higher rates of morbidity and complications.

I discuss the increased risk of postoperative pulmonary problems, including, but not limited to those discussed elsewhere, as well as skin loss or necrosis, bruising, bleeding, flap impairment, delayed wound healing, scarring, and incisional alopecia effects that could be permanent and significantly compromise the outcome of the procedure.

I discuss seeking the benefits of a professional counselor, if needed, to stop smoking. I also informed the patient that nicotine substitutes, such as inhalers, patches, and gums, are unacceptable in the perioperative period and that these drugs and devices also impair wound healing.

I ask my patients to sign an informed consent form acknowledging that they understand the risks of smoking relative to facial surgery.

GLOSSARY OF TERMS

throughout this book there have been many medical and procedural terms used to describe procedures and processes. We have created this simple and useful glossary in order to help you quickly understand some of these terms.

Acne: A common skin condition characterized by the excess production of oil from sebaceous glands in which the hair follicles become plugged and pimples form. This condition most frequently occurs during the teenage years and is also common in mid-adulthood as hormone levels change.

Acne scars: A consequence of acne. The scars range from pits, grooves to a wavy and undulating irregular appearance.

Alopecia: The loss of hair either in a region or extensive in nature. Hair loss or alopecia may accompany incisions made in hair bearing regions.

Banding: Caused by aging, these are vertical bands of excess skin in the neck. Banding could also be caused by excess or stretched muscle.

Blepharoplasty: Cosmetic procedure involving the skin and muscles around the eyes. Commonly referred to as an eyelid lift, this procedure works to correct the sagging, bulging, or loose skin and fat deposits that can develop around the eyes.

Botox: This is an injectable that is made from the botulinum toxin. It is used to stop the nerve response from the muscles to smooth out lines and wrinkles. Most often used to treat forehead lines, crow's feet, and lines around the mouth, this is a temporary treatment that needs to be repeated every few months. Similar to Dysport and Xeomin.

Botulinum toxin: The generic term for the Botox, Xeomin and Dysport injectable muscle relaxer and its derivative.

Browlift: Cosmetic procedure to adjust the skin around the eyes and forehead. This is most often an endoscopic procedure where the eyebrows are elevated to reduce wrinkling.

Canula: A small surgical instrument that is used for liposuction procedure to loosen the fat cells and remove them from the body.

Cheiloplasty: Cosmetic procedure to reduce or augment the lips.

Chemexfoliation: See chemical peel below.

Chemical peel: Cosmetic procedure to remove the upper layers of skin with a chemical solution. There are several strengths of solution available and each offer its own results.

Cheek augmentation: Cosmetic procedure to change the cheeks, also referred to as malarplasty.

Chin augmentation: Cosmetic procedure to change the size or shape of the chin and jaw line, also referred to as genioplasty.

Closed rhinoplasty: Cosmetic procedure on the nose where incisions are made inside of the nasal passages. It is an alternative approach to open rhinoplasty.

Collagen: This is the building block of the skin, cartilage, connective tissues, and bone. It is a major component of the body and it also used on fillers to plump areas of the face and body.

Coronal forehead lift: Specific cosmetic procedure that is used for a brow lift. It describes the incisions that are made ear to ear, over the top of the head. Previously a common technique for forehead and brow rejuvenation, it is considered outdated by some surgeons.

Crows Feet: The fine lines and wrinkles that form around the eyes. They are often caused by sun exposure. Smoking contributes to their formation. Smiling and facial motion also imprints lines upon this region.

Deep plane face lift: Specific cosmetic procedure that is used for a face lift. The incision site is below the superficial musculoaponeurotic system, allowing for not only the skin to be lifted, but the muscle and fascia as well.

Dermabrasion: Cosmetic procedure where fine sanding is used to smooth out the skin of the face. Top layers of skin are removed with a diamond tipped medical instrument.

Dermatitis: An inflammatory condition of the skin caused by an allergic reaction or contact with an irritant. Common symptoms include redness and itching.

Dermis: The middle layer of the skin lying beneath the epidermis. The dermis is a combination of blood vessels, hair follicles, and oil glands. Collagen and elastin create support within the dermis. Wrinkles occur within the dermal layer.

Deviated septum: A condition in which the partition that divides the nose it into two nostrils, the nasal septum, is crooked and obstructs nasal breathing. The condition is commonly treatable with surgery.

Dysport: This is an injectable that is made from the botulinum toxin. It is used to stop the nerve response from the muscles to smooth out lines and wrinkles. Most often used to treat forehead lines, crow's feet, and lines around the mouth, this is a temporary treatment that needs to be repeated every few months. Similar to Botox and Xeomin

Ear pinning: Cosmetic procedure of pulling the ears in closer to the face, this procedure is also called an otoplasty.

Elastin: A protein found with collagen in the dermis that gives structure and support to the skin and organs.

Endoscope: A small surgical instrument that serves as a telescope allowing surgeons to go into the body though smaller incision sites. This instrument allows for less invasive procedures to be performed.

Endoscope forehead lift: Cosmetic procedure using the endoscope to complete the forehead lift and remove wrinkles from the forehead.

Fndoscope midface lift: Cosmetic procedure using the endoscope to elevate the cheeks and midface region.

Exfoliate: To remove the top layers of skin. Chemical peel, dermabrasion and laser skin resurfacing are techniques in which the skin is exfoliated.

Eyelid lift: Cosmetic procedure where the skin, fatty tissue, and muscles around the eyes are tightened. This procedure is also called a blepharoplasty.

Facelift: Cosmetic procedure where the skin, fatty tissue, and muscles of the face are tightened to create a more youthful appearance. This procedure is also called a rhytidectomy.

Fascia: This is the non-elastic tissue that is just below the skin and above the muscles. It helps to keep the muscle system in place. In different cosmetic procedure this can be modified.

Fillers: Several different cosmetic substances that can be injected into the face in order to smooth out lines, wrinkles, and plump up areas that have started to fall flat.

Graft: Surgical process of moving tissue from one part of the area to another for reconstruction. This commonly happens during rhinoplasty procedures.

Hemangioma: A type of red or blue birthmark formed in the skin as a result of a concentration of small blood vessels. A variety of lasers may be used to treat hemangiomas.

Hooding: The descriptive term for sagging around the eyelids. This upper eyelid sagging can eventually obstruct vision.

Hyaluronic acid: A naturally occurring sugar that is widely distributed throughout the human body in connective tissues, skin and nerve tissue. Used as a basis for the soft tissue fillers in cosmetic surgery such as Juvederm, Restylane and Perlane.

Hyperpigmentation: A skin condition in which there is excessive pigmentation affecting the skin. Regions of hyperpigmentation appear darker than neighboring areas. Hyperpigmentation may be a result of sun exposure, prior surgery or the nature of the affected individual's skin type.

Hypertrophic scar: A raised and thickened red scar, similar to a keloid scar in appearance. Importantly, a hypertrophic scar remains within the boundaries of the injury site whereas a keloid scar grows and spreads.

Hypopigmentation: A skin condition in which there is a lack of pigmentation or lightening of a region of skin.

Implant: A piece of synthetic material that is used to create new shapes under the skin. Implants are often used to balance the appearance of the cheeks, chin, jowl region, jawline in facial plastic surgery.

Juvederm: This is a specific trade name for hyaluronic acid, which is used as cosmetic filler to increase and plump up specific areas of the face and to smooth crow's feet, lines around the mouth and to create fuller lips. Similar to Restylane.

Keloid scar: A type of scar that continues to grow beyond the initial site of an injury. This type of scar is caused by too much collagen forming while the skin is being repaired. Keloid scars grow in a crab-like fashion beyond the site of injury. The tendency to develop keloid scars is genetic and is most commonly seen in Native Americans, African Americans and Asians. Keloids rarely occur on the central face.

Keratin: This protein is the skin's main supporting material. Keratin also comprises hair and nails. Keratin makes skin rigid.

Laser: Cosmetic instrument that uses light amplification to treat the skin. This process makes it so the face can be changed without the need of incisions. There are many different kinds of lasers that are used for medical purposes including the removal of wrinkles, skin imperfections, growths, brown spots, spider veins and tattoos.

Lip Augmentation: A procedure done to improve deflated, drooping, or sagging lips, correct their symmetry, or reduce fine lines and wrinkles. Lip augmentation may be performed with a filler, an implant or through a surgical procedure that reconfigures the appearance and shape of the lips.

Liposuction: Cosmetic procedure where fat cells are removed from the body with a small instrument called a canula.

Marionette lines: The long vertical lines that run from the corners of the mouth down to the jowl or chin. Deep marionette appear with aging and respond to injectable fillers.

Melanocyte: A pigment producing cell found in the skin, hair, and eyes that gives them their color.

Mini facelift: Cosmetic procedure done to bring a more youthful appearance to the face. The mini version is done with smaller incisions and is often used for younger patients.

Nasal septum: The small part of cartilage that separates the two nostrils in the nose. The nasal septum is often deviated creating obstructed nasal breathing.

Nasolabial fold: The pair of skin folds that run from each side of the nose to the corners of the mouth. They separate the cheeks from the upper lip. Deep nasolabial folds are viewed as a sign of aging. Fillers or direct excision are common methods of improving this region.

Nose job: Cosmetic procedure where the size and shape of the nose of augmented. This procedure is also referred to as rhinoplasty.

Open rhinoplasty: Specific cosmetic procedure where the incisions are made around the nose and through the center of the nose allowing for better access to the underlying structure of the face. The incision is barely perceptible and many surgeons feel this approach allows for a more detailed and predictable approach to nasal contouring.

Otoplasty: The surgical procedure that corrects misshaped or protruding ears.

Perlane: Specific name of a filler made from hyaluronic acid. It is not permanent filler, but it is longer lasting than other hyaluronic fillers such as Juvederm and Restylane. Because it is thicker and more dense than other hyaluronic acid fillers, it is often used for deeper folds and lines.

Photo-aging: The skin changes that occur due to sun exposure such as wrinkles and age spots.

Platysma: Name of the two broad muscles that run along the side of the neck.

Ptosis: The drooping of a body part. In facial plastic surgery, most commonly eyelid ptosis.

Radiesse: A volumizing soft tissue filler made from calcium-based microspheres and gel. It acts as a scaffold under the skin, providing structure plumpling lines and wrinkles. Radiesse is often used in the nasolabial foldes and labiomental creases.

Restylane: Specific name of a filler made from hyaluronic acid. It is not permanent filler, but it is often used to lessen lines around the mouth and plump the lips. Similar to Juvederm.

Rhinoplasty: Cosmetic procedure to change the size and shape of the nose. This procedure is often combined with septoplasty to improve nasal and sinus function while also improving the appearance of the nose.

Rhytid: Medical term for a facial wrinkle.

Rhytidectomy: Cosmetic procedure where the wrinkles and fine lines of the face are removed by pulling the skin tighter. This is also referred to as a facelift.

Rosacea: A skin disorder characterized by redness and puffiness on several areas of the face that include the cheeks and nose. Rosacea cannot be cured, but numerous treatments improve the condition over time.

Sallowness: A term used to describe a yellowish color of the skin seen with aging.

Sebaceous glands: The glands of the skin that secrete oil.

Spider vein: A vein that can be seen through the surface of the skin.

Stratum corneum: The outermost layer of the epidermis that creates a barrier with the outside world.

Subcutaneous: A term referring to the layer beneath the skin. The subcutaneous layer is comprised of fat, blood vessels and nerves.

Sun protection factor: Commonly seen on sunblock ingredients as "SPF." The sun protection factor is the amount of protection a suntan product provides. The higher the SPF, the greater the protection. An SPF of 15, for example, means that you can stay in the sun 15 times longer than without the Sunblock.

Suture: Stitches placed by a surgeon to hold tissue together or to close a wound.

Transconjunctival blepharoplasty: Specific cosmetic procedure where the skin, muscle, and fatty tissue around the eyes are tightened; also called an eyelid lift. In this version of the procedure the incision is made inside the lower eyelid so that an external skin incision is not neccesary.

Wattle: Descriptive word referred to a sagging neck line, mainly caused by excess skin and excess fat.

Xeomin: This is an injectable that is made from the botulinum toxin. It is used to stop the nerve response from the muscles to smooth out lines and wrinkles. Most often used to treat forehead lines, crow's feet, and lines around the mouth, this is a temporary treatment that needs to be repeated every few months. Similar to Botox and Dysport.

TESTIMONIALS OF
CLEVENS FACE AND
BODY SPECIALISTS

The following pages contain testimonials from recent patients of Dr. Clevens and Clevens Face and Body Specialists and Imagine MediSpa in Melbourne, Merritt Island and Suntree, Florida. The testimonials and information provided represent the personal experiences of the individual patients and are reprinted here for informational purposes only and each patient's own experience is variable. The information is provided on an as-is basis and in some instances certain elements of the experiences may have been altered to protect patient confidentiality.

Alaina, a 56 year-old Surgical Technologist from Reno, Nevada

About first stepping into Dr. Clevens' office ...

"Even just bringing myself to the clinic for the first time was a great challenge. I had done all of my homework. Hour after hour I would research the backgrounds of plastic surgeons – but to actually go to the clinic and talk to somebody about my issue was very difficult for me. When I finally did start going to clinics, I never felt right. I would have to wait for a considerable length of time, or I wouldn't feel very comfortable with the staff members. I even went to Los Angeles and consulted with some of the plastic surgeons of the stars. But what an experience that was. They made me feel like 'cattle' – get in and get out as fast as possible. When I heard about Dr. Clevens through a friend of mine here in Florida, I thought I'd give him a try. Again, as I said before, just getting into the center was a great challenge for me, but I made myself do it. My first visit was an eye-opener. I was impressed with the look of the office, and the staff was very friendly and accommodating. In my first visit I was surprised that I didn't meet with the surgeon, Dr. Clevens. I was expecting to, but the staff that I did meet with spoke to me like a real person – woman to woman – on my level. I felt comfortable and assured that I was doing the right thing. I was so impressed that I couldn't wait for my second visit and actually meet Dr. Clevens."

Naomi, a 44 year old executive secretary with a Fortune 500 company from Melbourne, Florida

After a 'Weekend Necklift' with Dr. Clevens...

"The very same afternoon after my weekend necklift with Dr. Clevens, I went about my routine chores around the house. I was really surprised that I had all this energy. I also found it quite strange because I was expecting a lot of pain. But, I didn't even have to take a Tylenol. Very surprised!"

M.J., a 42 year old marketing representative from Orlando, Florida

On learning about Dr. Clevens...

"I heard about Dr. Clevens only through research I had done on the internet. Being new in town, I didn't know anybody; but Dr. Clevens' website looked convincing. When I contacted the office by phone, I was somewhat taken aback by the friendly tone of the speaker. I was also very surprised that they could see me in just a day or two. I liked that. When I was received by Shannon, the Patient Care Consultant, she was very knowledgeable and informative. I felt very comfortable with her because she actually listened to me and acknowledged what I wanted. She showed me pictures and explained various procedures. She informed me in a very professional manner just exactly what needed to be done. The whole staff at the center seemed very professional and organized. Feeling at ease, it was easy for me to make my decisions."

Jackie, a 40 year old travel agent from Deerfield Beach, Florida

Thoughts about a facelift, an eye lift and a full-face laser skin resurfacing procedure with Dr. Clevens...

"Out of all the internet searches I had done on plastic surgeons, Dr. Clevens had perfect stars from all of his patients. They had no complaints at all. So, why would I not consider him? I immediately got on the phone and called. I was very nervous with my first phone call to The Clevens Center – I don't know why, but I just was. But, the lady on the phone was so nice; it was as if we had known each other for a long time, so I was relieved."

Carol, a 38 year old mother of three who had recently relocated to Florida from Tennessee.

On first meeting Dr. Clevens and his team...

"My first encounter with Dr. Clevens was truly amazing. I was expecting a rather cold, scientific person with a matter-of-fact personality. However, nothing could be further from the truth. Dr. Clevens approached me with a very warm and person-able demeanor. What struck me the most was that he spoke to me and not at me. He put me at ease immediately, as if we were already mutual friends. He called me by my first name and made me feel important, as if I were the only one in the world being treated – very unlike my Los Angeles experience. I was also really impressed by the fact that Dr. Clevens only works on faces and nothing else. That says some-thing to me – a type of reassurance. I have a friend who had facial surgery done by a general doctor: She never felt right about the process and the results were very disappointing for her. I felt Dr. Clevens' expertise and knowledge was so impressive that when I left his office I had no doubt that I was with the right doctor. I was also very excited that I had actually found a person, after all my searching, that had gen-uinely listened to my concerns and actually acknowledged what I was saying. When I left the office after our meeting, I felt good, connected, respected, and safe. My first visit with him truly exceeded my expectations."

Beth, a 49 year old retail executive from Los Angeles, California

About Laser Skin Resurfacing with Dr. Clevens...

"I would like to give Dr. Clevens my compliments and I want my experience to spread out to other people in order to know him more and more. I really believe that different doctors make different outcomes and I am so proud of Dr. Clevens. I have had Laser Resurfacing to get rid of acne scars and they went from 70% to 80% gone so far. I have four more times to go and it's just amazing. The scar has gone away. Before it was deeper…now it's shallower and almost gone. You can see the difference every time he does it. He is knowledgeable, thoughtful and cares about what your concerns are…and he makes you look better. I thank his work for that. I'm really, really happy!!!"

Cindy, a 46 year old beautician from Suntree, Florida

About Dr. Clevens and his charitable work in Africa...

"I knew I wanted to come to Dr. Clevens because I've had friends who recommended him and another doctor recommended him to me. He is such a regular guy and he makes me feel so relaxed. I love reading about his professional occupation- that he has gone to Africa to help the children over there and he has been interested in helping people who need it. And he runs a very well organized office, unlike a lot of other doctors' offices. I really like that and I was very impressed with every single person I have met there. I probably have to see Dr. Clevens for a couple more months before I can fully see the results of the blepharoplasty and laser surgery I had under my eyes, but I'm sure I will be very happy with the ending result."

Alice, a 52 year old hospital administrator from Rockledge, Florida

About Dr. Clevens and his experience with Botox and fillers...

"I've lived in the Melbourne, FL area for sometime and have been familiar with Dr. Clevens. I follow along with his different articles and seminars I've been to. I'm very impressed by his education so my first thought when I wanted Botox and fillers was to go see him. He is a great person to sit and talk with and he's straight up. I explained what my concerns were and Dr. Clevens had so many thoughts to give. His assistant is great as well. They explained everything prior to my procedures and it was not uncomfortable at all. I also had Restylane in my lips. I thought they were very good preparing for everything and the outcome was great."

Lilly, a 38 year old pharmaceutical representative from Orlando, Florida

Thoughts about a late night check up call from Dr. Clevens...

"One thing that surprised me," she enthusiastically says, *"was that the night before the surgery, Dr. Clevens called me and asked if I had any fears or any questions. He also called me the night immediately after the surgery to find out how I was feeling – I have never had a doctor, not to mention a surgeon, call me personally and ask how I was after a procedure. This was something special. Dr. Clevens made me feel that I was important. He was genuinely concerned about my welfare."*

Katie, a 44 year old golf professional from Sydney, Australia

On receiving a house call from Dr. Clevens…

"Well, on the day of the surgery," he begins, "I felt safe and confident in Dr. Clevens' skills. I felt very secure because Dr. Clevens and his staff gave me a great feeling of self-assuredness – confirming that this was really what I wanted to do. They all comforted me – I felt absolutely no pain whatsoever. And to top it off, Dr. Clevens came and visited me the very next day after I had returned home – on a Saturday! I felt honored that he would do this for me."

Natania, a 55 year old clothing designer from Long Island, New York

Comments on the day of surgery with Dr. Clevens…

"On the day of the surgery," she explains, "I noticed that the nurses were all in a good mood. They were smiling and laughing… I wasn't nervous at all. There's something in smiles that is reassuring and relieving. I figured, if the people that are taking care of me are happy and content, then I should be, too. Shannon, the Surgical Nurse, came in and sat next to me. She held my hand and rubbed my back. She assured me that everything was going to be alright. Now that right there was tranquilizing in itself. Oh, and when Dr. Clevens came in, that just did it! Dr. Clevens has a way of calming you. He made me feel very relaxed. No wonder he got such high ratings all throughout my internet search. With all the other surgeons I looked at, Dr. Clevens was the only one that had perfect stars from all the patients that responded to survey questions about bedside manners. There were no complaints – not one. Knowing I was in such good care, I had no worries at all."

Stephanie, a 64 year old dance instructor from Barefoot Bay, Florida

On referral to Dr. Clevens by a dermatologist…

"My dermatologist, at a different practice, recommended Dr. Clevens. I had a Forehead Flap procedure in February of 2009. I had a skin cancer. He made me feel like he could close it up and make me look normal again. That's what I wanted. So, I trusted his words and everything. If you find yourself having skin cancer, do not worry because Dr. Clevens is here to fix you."

Lois, a 66 year old retired customer care representative from Cocoa, Florida

On recognizing cosmetic surgery as a motivation to quit smoking…

"Well, when Dr. Clevens told me I would have to stop smoking, caution lights went up all over the place. I had been smoking since I was a teenager – how was I going to quit just like that? I started out in my mind thinking that I wasn't going to smoke for only 2 weeks. But one thing led to another, and now I've been 2 years without a cigarette. I can't lie to you, every day the craving knocks on my door and I still want one. But I got to tell you, I sure feel a lot better. I can actually breathe without having to think about breathing. Plus, I don't have all that bad after-taste that can get kind of gross. Nor do I have that horrible morning cigarette breath. I'm not squinting anymore 'cause no smoke gets in my eyes – so that right there saves me a lot of wrinkles. And what's really nice is that I'm not coughing anymore, especially in the morning. What a relief! So, I truly got a double whammy here with Dr. Clevens. I got my nice facelift and bleph, looking like a million, and on top of that I feel a lot better. Why, I'd be willing to bet I added literally years to my life now that I don't smoke. The quality of life just seems a lot better now that I don't smoke. And, I got to tell you, my face? Absolutely tops! So, a new face and a better quality of life? It doesn't get any better than that! Thank you, Dr. Clevens – ten times over."

Dan , a 52 year old general contractor from Indialantic, Florida

About Dr. Clevens and his artistic talent…

"I interviewed with several doctors and what was most impressive about Dr. Clevens was all the before-and-after pictures he took to show all of the different angles of the face, and giving me the view of my face that I don't see. It was really interesting. Every other doctor I went to wanted to know what I wanted, while Dr. Clevens really sat down and said, "This is what I would like to do," and I felt he was more of an artist than the other doctors. I wound up having liposuction across my neck, chin implant, and injections around my mouth, in my lips and under my eyes. My favorite part about the results is having an actual neck. My friends see me and they want to have it done, too. Everything went very smoothly."

"If you are thinking about doing something, you shouldn't wait. You should go ahead and do it because it changes everything about you and your life, and it's really a nice feeling to have those final results and see the differences that you've wanted to have done. I think that's the most important."

Juan, a 29 year old rhinoplasty patient from Panama, Central America

About Mohs surgery and skin cancer care with Dr. Clevens…

"In October I had an eyelid surgery and a squamous cell carcinoma cut out, and more recently Sculptra treatments. I really like Dr. Clevens. I was referred by a dermatologist and she told me how nice he was. I had a positive attitude when I went in, but I just really like him as a person. He's very talented and I respect his work and his professionalism. He removed the squamous cell out of my lip and it came out well in the end, so I'm thankful for that. I'm happy with my eyes as well because they are natural. No one has even noticed that I had an eyelid surgery."

Anne, a 72 year old retired bookkeeper from Egypt Park, Florida

On the surgery center experience...

"I underwent an endoscopic browlift and upper eyelid lift and on the day of my procedure, I did sense quite a bit of anxiety; however, once I got to the facility, all of the staff really gave me a lot of assurance. I then felt really comfortable going into the O.R. During recovery I also felt comfortable. The staff continued to watch me carefully and they were all easily accessible. They were always very polite and professional."

Lance, a 51 year old cruise ship executive from Windermere, Florida

Thoughts about eyelid surgery to improve vision …

"Before surgery," she relates, *"I had to literally tape my eyelids back in order to see right. Not only that, but I was also very self-conscious of people looking at me and seeing my drooping eyelids. Now I know that not everybody goes around looking at peoples' eyelids, but it got to the point where I couldn't even talk to my friends without thinking about it. Now that I've had my surgery, my eyes are perfect! My eyelids are no longer blocking my vision and I no longer think that people are looking at them. Most importantly, now I can read, even late at night, and I can see just perfectly. Really, my operation has literally changed the way I see things. Catch my drift?*

Martha, a 62 year old school teacher from St. Cloud, Florida

About the Weekend Necklift™ by Dr. Clevens…

"Dr. Clevens had done a small procedure for me before I got the Weekend Necklift and he had done a procedure for my husband, too, so he has a great reputation from my personal experiences. I was thrilled when I qualified for a Weekend Necklift when he told me that I didn't need a Facelift. I needed to do a small office follow up in order to get it right. Dr. Clevens agreed that the initial result did not meet his expectations and asked me if I was interested in doing some further work. I said "yes" as long as it's of no cost to me, and he didn't hesitate. He said, "Don't worry, we'll get it right." Everybody heals differently, and he did in fact get it right. He's a very competent doctor."

Marie, a 47 year old college counselor from Kissimmee, Florida

Another doctor's impression of Dr. Clevens …

"I would definitely recommend Dr. Clevens, without a doubt. I am a doctor myself and Dr. Clevens has good reviews from other colleagues and within the community. The consultation was very comprehensive and detailed, and I felt I was in good hands. Everything from the Septorhinoplasty went smoothly and as expected. There is a definite improvement in my overall look and I feel more confident, so I am very pleased with everything."

Synthia, a 61 year old college admissions counselor from Amethyst, North Carolina

On professionalism among the staff of Clevens Face and Body Specialists…

"I found the consultation with Dr. Clevens to be extremely professional, pleasant, and not intrusive at all. He was easy to talk to. His staff was informative and pleasant. The procedure was well explained with clear directions as far as what to expect. The results from the upper and lower blepharoplasty have been excellent! The scarring is at a minimum, if you can even see anything at all. I'm extremely happy."

Jim, a 42 year old internist from Satellite Beach, Florida

About a complete facelift with Dr. Clevens…

"A friend of my cousin's had Blepharoplasty done with Dr. Clevens, and was very pleased with the results. I did research online and he seemed liked an excellent choice. I underwent a complete Facelift five weeks ago plus a CO2 laser on the entire face through the care of Dr. Clevens and his staff. I accidentally came in on the wrong day for my consultation. It wasn't scheduled until the week after but Dr. Clevens was nice enough to get me in that very same day. The preoperative consultation done by nurse Kim was excellent. She did a fabulous job. She's been a great nurse the entire time that I've spent with her. And Dr. Clevens did an amazing job with the surgery. We'd had a couple of miscommunications about the number of cleansings to do to the face and I did have a side effect of an earache which the doctor attended to. And by coming in that often, we ended up figuring out that I was cleansing my face too much one week and I had to limit it to about a few times weekly instead of five or six. That was the one main problem. Other than that, everything has healed nicely and the aesthetician has given excellent advice and it's been a good experience. Now I am amazed and I couldn't be more pleased with the excellent results, and they're not even final. "

Francesca, a 62 year old restauranteur from Belle Haven, Connecticut

After eyelid surgery with Dr. Clevens…

"A friend told me about Dr. Clevens' work. She knew a couple of people who had Upper Blepharoplasty surgery with him. Since I was interested in the same eyelid surgery, I went to see Dr. Clevens. Our meeting was very good, very informative and everybody working there was professional, yet friendly. He answered all of my questions about the procedure. Even after our meeting I would just call in my questions. I went in for my scheduled Upper Eyelid surgery on June 21st at the surgery center Dr. Clevens works out of, and found the entire staff to be wonderful. Following the surgery, I had expected a bit more pain, but I had none and the recovery was very easy. It has not yet been a full month since my surgery, but I already notice very much of a difference. I would definitely suggest Dr. Clevens as your facial plastic surgeon."

Ray, a 52 year old graphic designer from Cocoa Beach, Florida

Back to golf soon after facelift and necklift with Dr. Clevens…

"I had a Facelift and a neck and eye procedure on June 5th, just over a month ago. I'm back to playing golf and life is normal again. I came to Dr. Clevens because my husband had some work done and the ladies that I played golf had mentioned his name. He and the staff's professionalism added to my decision. Tammy did an excellent presentation for me prior to the procedures. During the consultation, they take a lot of time with you. You certainly never feel rushed. You can understand how they get backed up because I never at any time felt rushed. They were certainly willing to answer all my questions and Tammy is very knowledgeable. I couldn't be more pleased with the results. Most of the swelling and bruising is gone and it's everything that I expected. He was conservative and that's what I like because I don't look like I've been in the wind tunnel. With the amount of work that I had, I don't know that I was ready for care that it was going to take. My husband did a wonderful job, but I think people need to be aware that they just can't do it on their own. During the process, I got to see Kim a lot after the surgery and she is wonderful. I would highly recommend her and Dr. Clevens. I've already told people to come see him."

Marsha, a 59 year old retired dermatology nurse from Stuart, Florida

Some comments on Dr. Clevens' reputation in Central Florida…

"I knew some folks that had gone to see Dr. Clevens, and he has a very good reputation in Central Florida, so he was a natural choice for me for a blepharoplasty and facelift. He gave some suggestions and there were some things he suggested that I chose not to do, so he was very open about what could be done and what the outcome would be. One of the things I liked is that he is very diversified. He has a private practice, but he also has a life, too. I think that makes him more real to his patients."

Karen, a 44 year old homemaker from Tampa, Florida

On injectables and Botox at Clevens Face and Body Specialists

"I've had a few procedures done with Dr. Clevens. I've had injectables and Botox. I had Botox done in March of this year, and I just had more injectables of Radiesse today. What stands out the most to me is that he takes time and listens to what my concerns are. I look five years younger, which is pretty good."

Kim, a 42 year old model from Celebration, Florida

On Artisan skin resurfacing and hemangioma treatment with Dr. Clevens

"I've had three Artisan Treatments over the last six months, at the Clevens Center. I also had a Facial Laser about 12 years ago with Dr. Clevens. I came in most recently to have a hemangioma on my cheek treated. Then, I decided to have the whole face lasered for cosmetic reasons, to improve both skin elasticity and fine wrinkles. I saw the results a week after the procedure. It's a very efficient, well-run office."

Annie, a 56 year old retired sheriff's deputy from Queen's, New York

Some kind sentiments about our practice...

"My first trip to the office was the same type of experience – like I had known everybody for a long time. Now, every time I come to the center, it's like I'm just with a bunch of my girlfriends. I really didn't know what to expect with my first visit with the doctor himself, but once I met him I immediately felt comfortable. Dr. Clevens seemed very relaxed and that made me feel relaxed. He has this way of calming you, you know what I mean? I told him about my reasons for coming, and he listened closely, like he was extremely interested in what I had to say. I told him that when my husband died in 2008, the experience was really draining on me and it had manifested itself on my face. Everything on my face was droopy and sad looking. It was as if my husband's death was weighing on me so much, and my facial skin was taking that weight – I couldn't believe it!"

Jahnelle, a 58 year old nurse from Cocoa, Florida

A man's viewpoint about his cosmetic surgery experience at The Clevens Center...

"I was reluctant to come into a plastic surgeon's office at first. When Dr. Clevens said that he could help me and that my concerns were similar to that he heard from other men, I was ecstatic. When we went over the video imaging pictures and he showed me what could be done, I gained a new confidence. He made me feel positive and he made me feel good about myself. I think this is extremely important when choosing the right facial plastic surgeon. I've had a lot of duty stations in the Army and, I mean, you hear so many different horror stories about this type of thing, like people going down to Mexico to save money but coming back with bad jobs on their faces and things like that. I think you really have to be careful. I feel that I was careful. I had done my homework. I had followed the advice of my primary physician, I had done the research, and I had talked to my friends and neighbors who know Dr. Clevens and his work, all of whom had great comments about him. After my first two sessions at the clinic, I felt relaxed, courageous and self-assured."

Robert, a 64 year old retired Army Colonel from Bozeman, Montana

After an endoscopic browlift and an upper eyelid lift with Dr. Clevens...

"After an endoscopic browlift and an upper eyelid lift withry is that he does so much community service. To me, this says a lot about the man. It shows that he is dedicated to people and he is concerned about their well-being. I mean, nobody wants a jerk operating on something as important as your face, right? I also really liked the fact that he is a humanitarian. His trips to Africa to help those people speak volumes! I mean, he doesn't have to do that – it's just the way he is. He truly wants to help people."

Dave, a 56 year old architect from Melbourne Beach, Florida

On Dr. Clevens and his candor...

"Dr. Clevens was very straightforward with his explanations. He explained every-thing in a down-to-earth manner. Being so informative, he took away all of my fears."

Katie, a 32 year old personal trainer from Vero Beach, Florida

On a quicker than expected recovery after a Direct Necklift with Dr. Clevens...

"I was really surprised; my recovery time was much shorter than I had arranged for. I was actually doing paperwork the very next day." Although any kind of physical work in excess immediately after surgery is strongly discouraged by any facial plastic surgeon, don't let the excitement of a successful operation get the best of you."

Dr. Larry, a retired 68 year old family physician from Harpswell, Maine

On a longer than expected recovery after surgery with Dr. Clevens...

"Actually, my recovery has taken longer than I expected. I'm ten weeks out and I'm still having some swelling around the ears. I kind of anticipated that – but just not so long." Synthia goes on to offer very valuable words of wisdom when she adds, "I think everyone should hire a private nurse for recovery. My husband was really overwhelmed by the operation and my recovery time. He had to do a lot of things around the house by himself that I usually take care of. It's so surprising what is tak-en for granted. He wasn't used to that, nor did he know the details of the post-oper-ative treatment. This is where a private nurse would really come in handy. I would recommend having a private nurse to anyone having plastic surgery."

Heather, a 42 year old accountant from Belmont, Massachusetts

A returning patient's thoughts on Dr. Clevens…

"I had a procedure with Dr. Clevens 10 years ago and I thought he did very good work then…and 10 years later I decided to choose him again. I was actually going to have a third procedure done, but when this facelift was completed, the third one didn't have to be done. I wasn't pushed to do it either. They told me if I didn't want to do it that was perfectly all right and as far as I wanted to go was fine. Other offices, they would tell you that you don't want to do it; but no, not here."

"I think Dr. Clevens has gotten better with his experience from doing facelifts so often. I'm very happy, and if my family or close friends want plastic surgery, I will tell them to go to Dr. Clevens."

Joy, 62 year old school teacher from the Abaco, Bahamas

On Dr. Clevens' professionalism…

"I've had very good experiences with Dr. Clevens. On July 1st I had a Facelift. I've had procedures before and I've always found him to be very nice and professional. I certainly will recommend him to others. He is an excellent surgeon."

Cheryl, a 56 year old newspaper editor from Toledo, Ohio

On laser skin resurfacing with Dr. Clevens...

"Dr. Clevens not only makes you feel comfortable, but he also gives the impression that he sincerely wants to do something for you. When you first walk into his office to talk with him, it's a non-intimidating environment – very relaxing. He has a very warm personality along with a great sense of humor – yes, a sense of humor – something I never would have thought a doctor with such an incredible background would have. And finally, I felt very confident and self- assured that Dr. Clevens is a facial plastic surgery specialist. I mean, if you are considering work done on your face, why would anybody go someplace else? To me, it's just a no-brainer."

CLEVENS FACE AND BODY
BEFORE & AFTER GALLERY

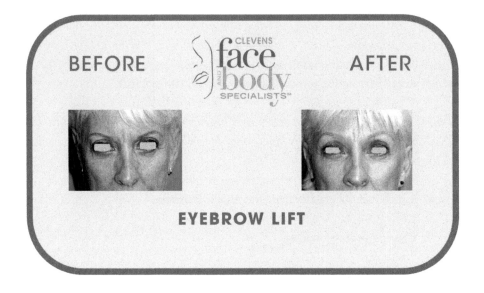

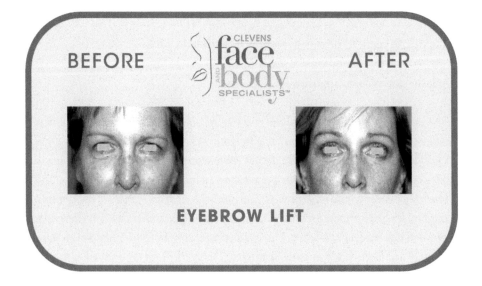

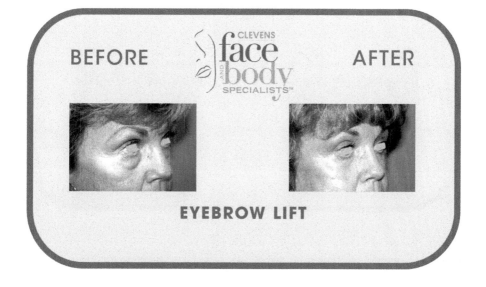

BEFORE AFTER

EYEBROW LIFT

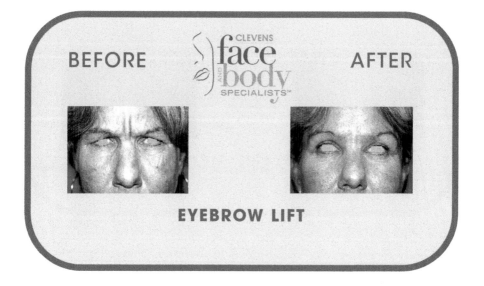

BEFORE AFTER

EYEBROW LIFT

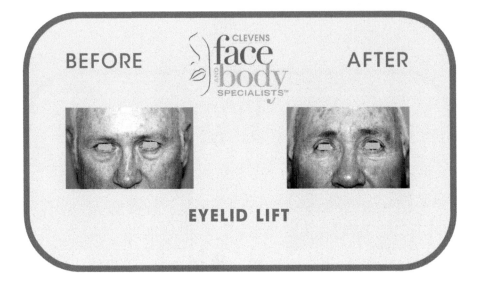

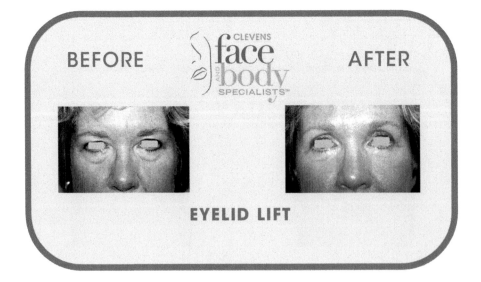

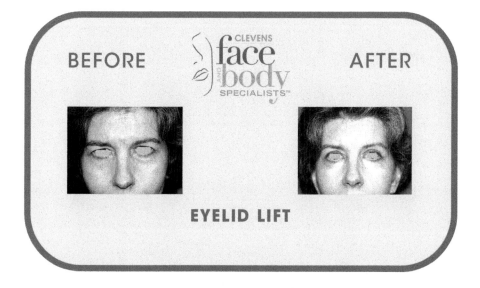

BEFORE · AFTER

EYELID LIFT

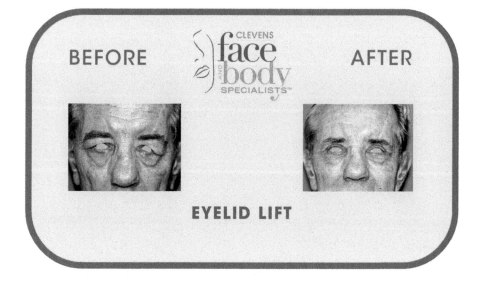

BEFORE · AFTER

EYELID LIFT

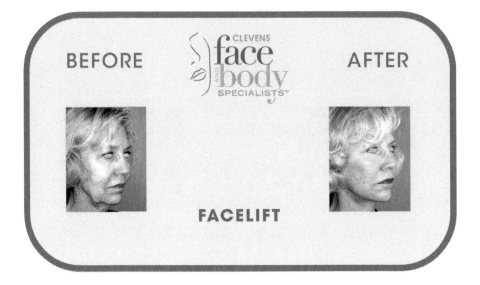

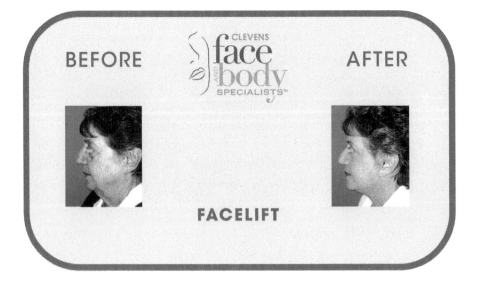

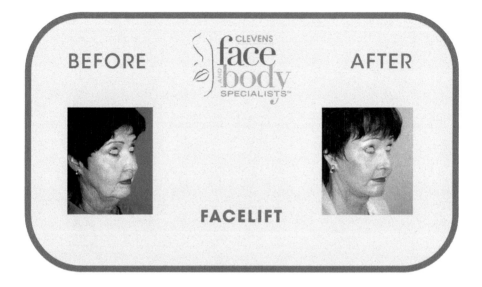

BEFORE

AFTER

FACELIFT

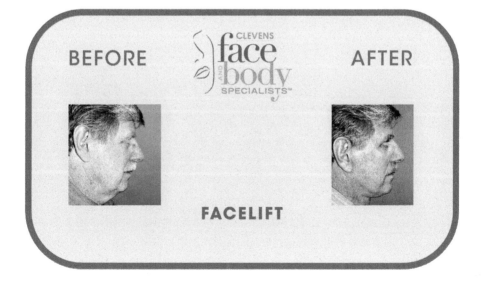

BEFORE

AFTER

FACELIFT

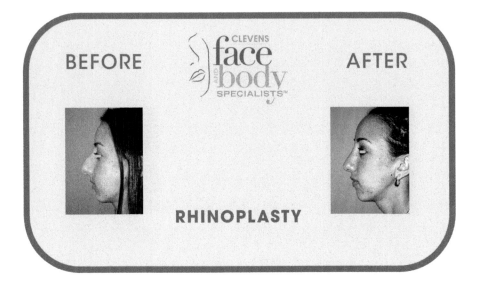

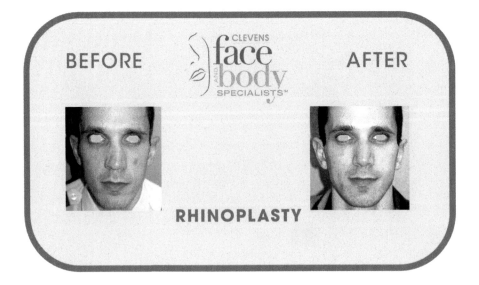

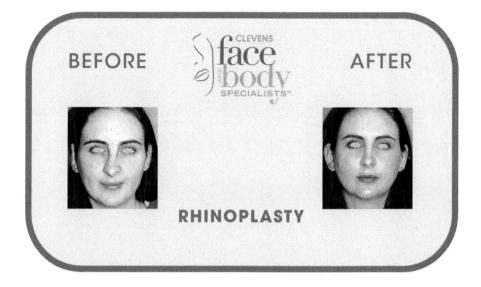

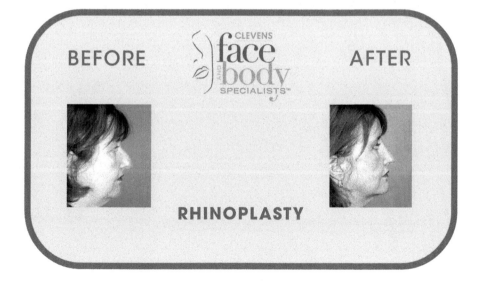

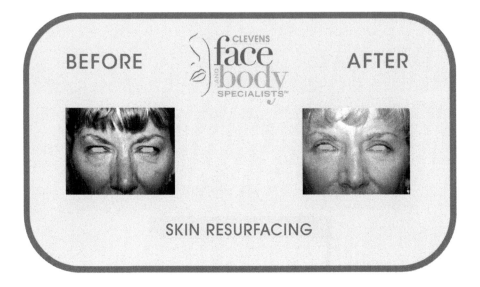

SKIN RESURFACING

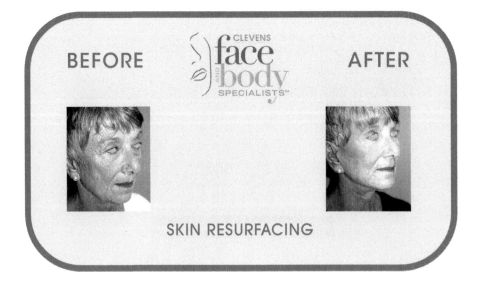

SKIN RESURFACING

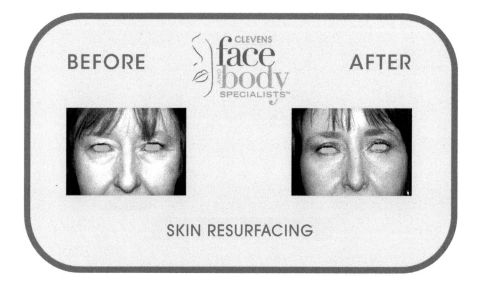

BEFORE

AFTER

SKIN RESURFACING

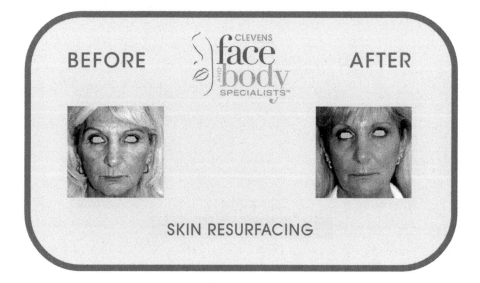

BEFORE

AFTER

SKIN RESURFACING

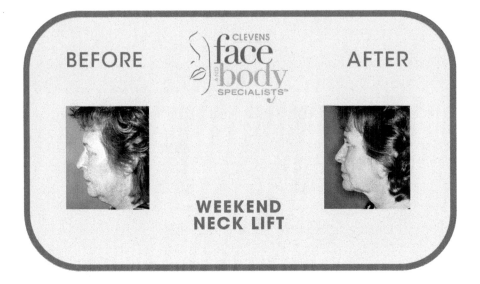

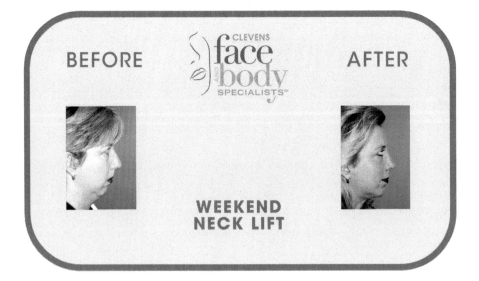